THE CLINICAL AUDIT HANDBOOK

improving the quality of health care

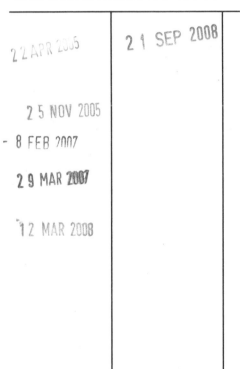

For Baillière Tindall:
Senior Commissioning Editor: Jacqueline Curthoys
Project Controller: Derek Robertson

THE CLINICAL AUDIT HANDBOOK

improving the quality of health care

Clare Morrell RGN BN RSCN MSc
Research and Development Officer (Clinical Audit),
Royal College of Nursing Institute, Oxford, UK

Gill Harvey RGN BNurs RHV DN PhD
Head of Quality Improvement,
Royal College of Nursing Institute, Oxford, UK

Foreword by
Professor Alison Kitson RGN BSc(Hons) DPhil FRCN
Director, Royal College of Nursing Institute

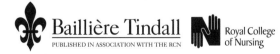

Baillière Tindall
PUBLISHED IN ASSOCIATION WITH THE RCN

Royal College
of Nursing

BAILLIÈRE TINDALL
An imprint of Harcourt Publishers Limited

© Harcourt Brace and Company Limited 1999
© Harcourt Publishers Limited 2001

✤ is a registered trademark of Harcourt Publishers Limited

First published 1999
Reprinted 2001

ISBN 07020 2418 X

British Library Cataloguing in Publication Data
A catalogue record for this book is available from the British Library

Library of Congress Cataloging in Publication Data
A catalog record for this book is available from the Library of Congress

The
publisher's
policy is to use
**paper manufactured
from sustainable forests**

Printed in China

Contents

Foreword

Over a decade of work and the experiences of many people have fashioned this book. It is the latest stage of the RCN Dynamic Quality Improvement Programme's development of key ideas around standards, quality and audit. And while it builds on the past, it seeks to make sense of the exciting changes around quality and audit that are upon us.

Reassuringly, those core principles of patient-centredness, ownership and local participation which were identified as the building blocks of the RCN's work on quality ('A framework for quality', 1989) are still centre stage. Indeed, with the introduction of clinical governance and the importance of local interpretation of national clinical guidelines to assure quality, the realisation of such concepts is all the more pressing.

This text will help clinical teams to make sense of their responsibilities around making audit a working part of their lives; not an optional extra, but an intrinsic part of everyday practice. It sets out in a clear way how we all can get involved and how we can celebrate our success. Importantly, it also shows how to involve consumers in routine audit.

For me this is a book that reflects the effort, character, spirit and optimism of many dear colleagues and friends – from those in the early days of the standard setting project in the RCN, to Clare Morrell and Gill Harvey, who have led the production of this latest work. Most especially, I would like to thank Helen Kendall whose innovative interpretation of Donabedian's structure, process and outcome concepts profoundly influenced the form and structure of the Dynamic Standard Setting System (DySSSy), the method developed to help nurses set standards and audit their care. And finally, a sincere acknowledgement to Avedis Donabedian himself for inspiring so many colleagues and helping us to ensure the challenge of quality improvement.

Professor Alison Kitson
Director, RCN Institute

Preface

This handbook has developed out of the Royal College of Nursing's work on quality and standards over the past twenty years, and specifically from the Dynamic Standard Setting System. Since 1985 the RCN has been promoting the use of local standard setting and audit as a means of quality improvement. In 1990 The Dynamic Standard Setting System, known as DySSSy, was published as a handbook[1], based on the experience of three years of running workshops. DySSSy was designed with the potential to be multi-professional and from the very first workshops nurses were encouraged to work toward this. In some areas nurses using DySSSy had always involved their colleagues from other professions and have naturally moved the system into an integral part of the clinical audit programme and quality strategy. Others, however, have found this transition difficult.

The idea for this handbook emerged from the recommendations of a recent evaluation[2] of the system which identified the need for explicit guidance in developing DySSSy for the multi-professional audience. The evaluation highlighted the changing health care agenda of recent years and showed how in places practitioners had been able to adapt the system to fit the changes in the structure and demands of the National Health Service.

The particular strengths of the DySSSy approach were the philosophy of improvement, the practice-led problem-solving approach and the emphasis on groups working together with a facilitator. These principles are entirely consistent with clinical audit as it is understood across health care. However, confusions around terminology, particularly the use of the term standard, have caused problems to the extent that programmes of quality improvement originally based on DySSSy have remained entirely separate from clinical audit activities in some areas. This handbook seeks to address those problems around terminology and brings DySSSy clearly within the present-day context of clinical audit.

The Royal College of Nursing is committed to promoting clinical effectiveness and has drawn up a comprehensive strategy to that end[3]. Clinical audit is seen as an integral part of that strategy, providing an important method for implementing national clinical guidelines and developing evidence-based practice.

This handbook can be used in a number of ways:

- *as a reference guide* for those already involved in clinical audit
- *as a learning resource* for individuals for self-directed study
- *as a project companion* for groups who are new to clinical audit and wish to use this as a flexible learning package.

Throughout the text 'time out' boxes are provided with suggestions for brief exercises to encourage reflection and learning. These are designed to be used by individuals or by groups. In addition, summaries are provided at the end of main sections as an aid to learning.

The handbook is set out in three parts. The first chapter introduces clinical audit and puts it in context with other related initiatives in health care. The second part, Chapters 2–5, provides a step-by-step guide to conducting a clinical audit project and the third part, Chapters 6–9, sets out the issues to be considered when implementing a clinical audit programme.

It is envisaged that having worked through this handbook you will be equipped with the necessary knowledge to design, plan and implement a clinical audit project together with your colleagues with a renewed enthusiasm for developing the quality of care to your patients.

Clare Morrell, Gill Harvey

References

1. RCN 1990 Quality patient care: the Dynamic Standard Setting System. Scutari, Harrow
2. Morrell C, Harvey G, Kitson AL 1995 The reality of practitioner based quality improvement, report no. 14. National Institute for Nursing, Oxford
3. RCN 1996 The Royal College of Nursing Clinical Effectiveness Initiative: a strategic framework. RCN, London

Acknowledgements

Thanks are due to members of the RCN Dynamic Quality Improvement Team past and present who have contributed to this book in the various formats in which much of the material has previously appeared, in particular Alison Kitson, Sophie Hyndman, Lesley Duff, Alison Loftus Hills, Elisabeth Morgan and Gabby Fennessy. We would also like to thank colleagues from the RCN Institute, especially Nicola Crichton and Sophie Staniszewska, for their advice and support.

Most importantly we would like to take the opportunity to thank the many patients, nurses and other professionals, especially the members of the DQI Network, who have been involved in shaping this work as it has evolved over the years. Particular thanks go to those who have contributed to this book by sharing their experiences in the form of examples to bring the theory to life.

1

What is clinical audit?

The essence of clinical audit is developing health care practice, something which practitioners have been attempting to do for generations. The quest to constantly develop our practice has aroused passions since the ancient world and it was the mission of Florence Nightingale:

> For us who Nurse, our Nursing is a thing which unless we are making *progress* every year, month, every week, take my word for it we are going *back*[1].

Florence Nightingale was a pioneer of systematic observation, standard setting and improvement of care. During the Crimean War at Scutari she realised that admission to the battle hospital increased a soldier's chances of death, so she set standards against which she measured practice. This process led to a drastic reduction in the rates of hospital-acquired infection and cut the mortality rate dramatically.

This first chapter begins by considering definitions of clinical audit and reasons for health care practitioners to get involved. Clinical audit conjures up different images for people. For some it is a fulfilling and enjoyable process of changing health care practice for the better. For others it appears to be only about collecting information and filling in a stream of pieces of paper for no apparent gain. It is hoped that by the time you have worked through this handbook you will see the potential that clinical audit has as a tool for improving patient care.

Although clinical audit might feel like a relatively new concept, the belief that clinical staff should be constantly seeking to improve care is as old as the professions themselves. You will have heard a variety of terms used to describe this process. In the nursing and therapy professions the term quality assurance has been used in the past which has been defined as 'deciding what should be, comparing what should be with reality, identifying the gaps and taking action'[2]. Quality assurance suggests that we are seeking to assure or provide a certain constant level of care. This handbook seeks to take that idea a step further and suggest that clinical audit needs to be seen as a means to continuous improvement – ensuring not just good care but an ongoing process of development; a journey that never ends.

This handbook aims to provide a map with which to navigate. Following this introductory chapter, Chapters 2 to 5 take you step by step through a process to undertake a clinical audit project. Chapter 6 then looks at some variations on the system and Chapters 7 to 9 examine the context of clinical audit in terms of the organisational approach necessary for a successful and integrated programme of clinical audit.

Defining clinical audit

The most commonly quoted definition of clinical audit is an adaptation of that originally put forward by the Department of Health[3], in working paper 6 (Medical Audit) of the White Paper 'Working for Patients', 1989:

> Clinical audit is the systematic and critical analysis of the quality of clinical care, including the procedures used for diagnosis, treatment and care, the associated use of resources and the resulting outcome and quality of life for the patient.

As clinical audit has been implemented across the UK it has come to be widely understood as a team approach to audit. This is reflected in the following definition which describes clinical audit as 'multi-disciplinary professional, patient focused audit, leading to cost-effective, high quality care delivery in clinical teams'[4]. The emphasis is on health care professionals working together to develop the quality of care received by patients.

In its 1994 publication, 'The evolution of clinical audit', the NHS Executive set out the fundamental principles associated with clinical audit which state that it should:

- be professionally led
- be seen as an educational process
- form a part of routine clinical practice
- be based on the setting of standards
- generate results that can be used to improve outcome of quality care
- involve management in both the process and outcome of audit

- be confidential at the individual patient/clinician level
- be informed by the views of patients/clients[3].

These principles include a whole range of issues you will need to consider when planning any clinical audit project and these are all addressed within the workbook. The list shows that clinical audit is not an isolated activity and it needs careful planning to be successful.

With the recognition of the importance of multi-professional teamwork in clinical audit came the broader question of who needs to be involved. This raised an awareness of the necessity to involve the consumers of the service – patients, carers and their representatives. This is explored in Chapter 7.

The developing profile of evidence-based medicine and clinical effectiveness has led to more recent policy statements from the NHS Executive emphasising the role that clinical audit has to play in clinical effectiveness, by getting research into practice.

> Clinical audit is and should remain a clinically led initiative which seeks to improve the quality and outcome of patient care through clinicians examining and modifying their practices according to standards of what could be achieved, based on the best evidence available (or authoritative expert opinion where no objective research-based evidence exists)[5].

To clarify what we mean by clinical audit, it is perhaps worth highlighting what clinical audit is not. Over the past few years there has been confusion about exactly what is and what is not clinical audit, compounded by the fact that across the UK all sorts of different projects have been allocated money from audit funds.

The Clinical Resource and Audit Group (CRAG) in Scotland set out what audit is not:

a. a system of ensuring that staff in training are making satisfactory progress, which is a function of professional educational bodies and Postgraduate Medical and Dental Education Committees
b. performance appraisal of posts in organisational terms, such as monitoring quantity of activity, time keeping etc.
c. a disciplinary mechanism
d. research, which is concerned with establishing new knowledge
e. needs assessment[6].

The Royal College of Speech and Language Therapists put it slightly differently. Audit is not:

- having a computer
- doing research
- finding fault in people's performance
- finding 'bad apples'
- checking up
- statistics
- 'top down' inspection[7].

Perhaps the best way of defining clinical audit is to illustrate it. The following example shows how clinical staff have worked together, gathered the best available evidence and acted over a period of years to improve care to patients.

Clinical audit of pressure area care

Wendy-Ling Relph, Practice Development Nurse, Royal Brompton Hospital

In October 1991, nurses and occupational therapists within Royal Brompton Hospital expressed concern about the provision of pressure-relieving devices for those identified as 'high risk' patients. In part, this was because of a prior publication stating that patients were inappropriately nursed on sophisticated pressure-relieving systems because their risk status was not reviewed regularly enough[8].

The development of a pressure sore means an increased hospital stay, increased discomfort and increased distress for the patient and their family. On further investigation it was found that once a pressure sore had formed, the cost implications were extremely high, with a grade 4 pressure sore, at the time, estimated as costing £25 000 to treat[9]. Additionally, this also meant an increased risk of costly litigation being instigated as, in 1991, health authorities were being sued anywhere between £100 000 and £1 000 000 by patients who had developed sores during their hospital stay. All of these reasons, including the findings that 95% of pressure sores are preventable[10], led to a clinical audit group for pressure area care being formed.

Although the treatment and prevention of pressure sores is seen by many as 'fundamental to the (nursing) profession's credibility as well as a searching test of its expertise'[11], the group has always recognised that it is a multi-professional issue with the causes being multifaceted.

As a result the group comprised nurses, occupational therapists, physiotherapists and dietitians. With the help of an experienced facilitator, all were involved in setting a standard and devising an audit tool.

As each member had expertise in different areas and all had much information to offer the group as a whole, it was important at the outset to ensure that everyone participated equally and each person's ideas and suggestions were discussed by the group in a non-hierarchical style. This was enabled by the facilitator. In order to achieve the aim of devising a hospital-wide standard and to ensure that the interest and motivation of each member was maintained, fortnightly meeting dates were set in advance. This allowed each member to plan and incorporate the meetings into their working schedule, ensuring that the group met on a regular basis.

Although each member was a representative for each of their wards and departments, it was important that the views and opinions of as many people as possible were incorporated. Therefore, between meetings, it was the responsibility of each member to discuss any new issues with their departmental teams and to feed back any suggestions and comments to the group. All relevant staff had the opportunity to comment upon the completed document before it was finally ratified. A review of the evidence was undertaken and where documented research evidence was not available, the consensus opinion of the expert group was utilised to decide upon current best practice.

The time taken from the raising of the first concerns through to completion of the objectives and criteria was 8 months. The pilot audit took place in June 1992. These results were used as a baseline for future developments and so a small convenience sample of 4 patients and 4 nurses were audited from each ward area.

The main findings were that 50% of the patient population were identified as at risk of developing a pressure sore, a number of mattresses were in poor condition and there was a lack of knowledge amongst ward nurses on areas related to pressure-relieving equipment. It was decided from this that a point prevalence study needed to be undertaken to give more specific information, particularly about how many of the total patient population suffered from pressure sores, their documented risk score and the state of each mattress within the hospital. A point prevalence study simply describes the number of people who have a pressure sore at a given point in time.

In addition, other standards were developed and issues explored as a result of the baseline data collected. It was highlighted both that the lack of lifting aids on the wards could be discouraging nurses from lifting and turning patients and that pain was likely to be a contributing factor as patients were prevented from moving in bed. As a result, clinical audit groups were set up for both of these areas (the pain project is presented in more detail in Chapter 4).

Over the years, representatives of the multi-professional teams involved have continued to meet. Unsurprisingly, few of the original group members work within the hospital in the same capacity as they did seven years ago. However, as group members have left, it has been their responsibility to identify someone to take their place and continue to develop their role.

Each year, the standard and the point prevalence study have been reviewed, re-audited and local and hospital-wide action plans devised to address new issues. These have included a mattress replacement programme and the writing of a policy to maintain this, identifying a nurse to coordinate both in-house and hired equipment and holding regular meetings with the link nurses to encourage information sharing.

The initial audit in 1992 identified the prevalence of pressure sores as being 19% of the patient population. This dropped dramatically over subsequent years and the 1997 results are just 3% of the patient population, within the DoH guidelines (1993)[12] stating a commitment to reduce the incidence of pressure sores in the NHS by 5%. The Trust's commissioners have taken a keen interest in the project and have adopted it as an outcome measure within the contracting process.

Why get involved?

Patient care reasons

As illustrated in the example above, the most pressing reasons for health professionals to get involved in clinical audit are the benefits to patients in terms of improved standards of care and the development of a more effective service. Clinical audit provides a systematic mechanism with which to do this and the opportunity to evaluate the results of any changes. The objective of clinical audit is to improve patient care by informing the health care professionals' understanding of their clinical practice[6].

Changes in health policy over the last decade have all emphasised the involvement of the public and individual patients in decisions about health care. The public is demanding that health services are seen to be implementing the findings of good research. With access to information technology there are increasing numbers of well informed patients. This emphasis on a consumer-led health service may also be contributing to the rise in complaints and litigation. All these factors strengthen the case for health professionals to be engaged in regular and systematic review of the treatments and services they provide.

Professional reasons

As professionals we constantly seek to develop our knowledge and skills in line with the latest available evidence. This has now become a requirement for most professional groups. Involvement in clinical audit can facilitate this process as teams work together to review and appraise the latest evidence in their field. Increasingly it is possible for clinical audit activities, particularly attendance at study days and conferences, to form an accredited part of continuing professional development.

The process of clinical audit is in itself a learning experience. Staff develop skills in audit methods and have the opportunity to further build working relationships within the multi-professional team.

Clinical audit provides valuable evidence of the effectiveness of professional roles. There are times when it can be helpful to demonstrate the professional contribution to patient care. As professionals we are responsible and accountable for our practice. Accountability demands that we can provide evidence of the standards of care that we provide.

Political reasons

There is a high level of interest in clinical audit and clinical effectiveness as a result of a number of factors including: the increasing costs of health care; increasing technology and complexity of health care; changing health needs of the population; and the increased emphasis on linking clinical and cost effectiveness. These issues feature prominently in recent health care legislation across the UK, particularly in the proposals to introduce national service standards, external quality monitoring and a statutory responsibility for health care quality, through the implementation of local clinical governance[13]. Clinical governance is defined as:

> ...a framework through which NHS organisations are accountable for continuously improving the quality of their services and safe-

guarding high standards of care by creating an environment in which excellence in clinical care will flourish[14].

In effect, clinical governance is an umbrella term for a range of activities that aim to maintain and improve standards of patient care. These include the following[15]:

- Systems for quality improvement, including clinical audit and evidence based practice.
- Systems for risk management and the management of performance, including critical incident reporting, clinical supervision and responding to patient complaints.
- Systems for ensuring accountability and responsibility for quality, for example, appointing a lead clinician for clinical governance and establishing a regular reporting system to the Chief Executive and management board.

These systems will need to be underpinned by an organisational culture that promotes a patient-focused approach to care, encourages multi-professional teamwork and enables open discussion about practice and learning from mistakes.

Clearly, clinical audit is an important component of clinical governance. At a political level, however, the emphasis is on making sure that clinical audit is an integral part of an overall organisation-wide approach to managing and improving the quality of patient care.

Why not get involved?

Time to commit to clinical audit activities is the major barrier to involvement[16]. Clinical audit has been criticised for taking staff away from clinical practice with very little to show for that investment. It has been pointed out that 'we should not accept uncritically what is urged upon us'[17]. It is therefore important to reflect upon whether this time can indeed be justified. It would appear that only if practice is being seen to develop, with clear evidence of improvements in patient care, can time out from practice really be considered worthwhile.

A note of caution, however: change takes time and clinical audit only provides a tool. Changing the attitudes which dictate the behaviour and practices of health professionals is a slow process and it may need months and years of persuasion before individuals are convinced of the need to do things differently.

What outcomes would you expect to see from clinical audit which would justify taking staff time away from clinical practice?

Summary

- Clinical audit is a dynamic process whose focus is improving patient care.
- It is a collaborative multi-professional activity.
- There are many reasons to get involved including political, professional and patient care factors.
- Clinical audit takes time.

Is clinical audit the right approach?

What is set out in the following chapters can be described as criterion-based audit, i.e. based on the development of specific criteria. You will come across a number of other methods of auditing practice and some of these are outlined in Chapter 6. Before embarking on a project it is worth considering what you are trying to achieve. You may have come across a problem in practice that requires a rapid response, a patient complaint or an adverse incident. Setting up a clinical audit project may not be the appropriate course of action.

In the past nurses have been keen to see standards written to cover the range of clinical practice issues. If staff are looking for guidance, it may be more appropriate to refer to a clinical

Table 1.1 **Approaches to solving clinical practice issues**

Problem	Solution
Need to determine best care for managing venous leg ulcers in the community	Get access to the Effective Health Care Bulletin on compression therapy for venous leg ulcers and the national clinical guideline which builds on this
Need to disseminate best practice to primary health care team	Distribute summary guides to all staff and adapt national guideline to a local clinical guideline or protocol
Need to implement and monitor local practice against best practice recommended in the guidelines	Establish a clinical audit project

procedure manual[18] or clinical guidelines. Table 1.1 sets out an example of where different documents may be useful.

Starting out with clinical audit

We have defined clinical audit and discussed reasons to get involved, so how do you begin? It may be useful to think of clinical audit as a cycle. This is very similar to the stages of practice development or action research with which you may be familiar. Various versions of the clinical audit cycle are in use across health care, but for our purposes the cycle consists of four main stages, as illustrated in Figure 1.1.

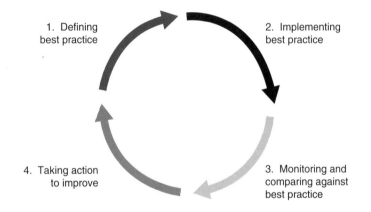

1. Defining best practice

2. Implementing best practice

4. Taking action to improve

3. Monitoring and comparing against best practice

Figure 1.1 **The four main stages of clinical audit.**

The process of clinical audit is set out in detail in the chapters that follow. *Defining best practice* is the subject of Chapter 2 – this involves deciding what best practice is. *Implementing the standard and preparing for monitoring* is the subject of Chapter 3. A tool for data collection is created and tested in practice. At the same time best practice is discussed with the team and plans made for implementation.

Monitoring and comparing the current situation with best practice is described in Chapter 4. A suitable sample is decided upon and data collectors prepared. Once the data have been collected they are compared against the standard and analysed appropriately.

With the data analysed, it is time to take stock and reflect with the clinical team. The next stage in the cycle is *taking action to improve*, which is the subject of Chapter 5. Staff need to take time to celebrate the success of their achievements, whilst action is agreed to improve the service in the areas where problems have been identified. Once the changes in practice have been made, monitoring takes place again to see whether things have improved.

Having completed the cycle, the group then considers whether it is possible to raise the standard to move further toward best practice. In this way quality improvement becomes an ongoing, continuous process, and the cycle can be more accurately visualised as a quality spiral.

It is important that clinical audit is not seen in isolation. Clinical teams working round the audit cycle need to link their activities to: (a) developments nationally in terms of policy and research and (b) systems within their organisation – communication channels and resources.

Clinical audit as a part of clinical effectiveness

Clinical audit needs to become a part of both clinical effectiveness and quality improvement. These ideas are discussed in more detail in Chapter 8. Clinical effectiveness can be seen as an umbrella term involving the implementation of evidence into clinical practice and the evaluation of that process. It therefore includes clinical audit, clinical guidelines and any other strategies used within the process. The RCN has defined clinical effectiveness as:

> applying the best available knowledge, derived from research, clinical expertise and patient preferences, to achieve optimum processes and outcomes of care for patients[19].

Clinical effectiveness has provided the opportunity to reflect upon what has been done in clinical audit and ensure that it incorporates the best available evidence and is carried out in a rigorous way.

There is sometimes a tension between local ownership and rigour. Some feel strongly that the important thing in clinical audit is that practitioners themselves are responsible for the process and that the methods used are of secondary importance – what is central to a project is building the team and encouraging new ideas. Others, however, point out that if the considerable resource of staff time is to be invested in a project it should be done well enough that its results can be trusted as the basis for changing practice, the emphasis being on the rigour of the method rather than the relationships within the team. The challenge is to develop a balance between the two.

The principles of clinical effectiveness can be applied to promote rigour in clinical audit using the following steps:

1. There is a clear stated reason for undertaking the audit, made explicit in the form of an objective.
2. Key stakeholders (professionals, patients, managers) are represented in the audit, according to the topic under study.
3. A systematic process is followed to derive the evidence base for objectives and criteria.
4. The objectives and criteria to be achieved are made explicit and reflect the available evidence.
5. There is an agreed process for disseminating and implementing the objectives and criteria.
6. Adequate and appropriate methods of sampling and data collection are employed to ensure representative audit findings.
7. There is an agreed method of comparing audit data against agreed objectives and criteria
8. A mechanism for feeding back audit data to participants is in place.
9. Solutions are discussed to address areas where objectives and criteria are not being achieved and a plan of action for improvement is agreed and implemented.
10. Re-audit is undertaken to determine where actions implemented have achieved the improvements planned.

Clinical audit within a framework for improvement

Clinical audit could be considered an internally applied mechanism for quality improvement as the control and ownership for clinical audit projects rests with the staff involved. Systems such as those produced by the International Standards Organisation, e.g. ISO 9000, or others, as described in Appendix 2, depend on inspection and might therefore be considered externally applied mechanisms for quality improvement.

A study of the implementation of three quality systems in nursing[20], two externally applied and one internally applied, concluded that ultimate success or failure depends not on the system itself but on the way in which a system is implemented and used. The study recommended that implementation takes place by devolving maximum control and ownership to practitioners. However, for this process to be successful, support and commitment must come from the top of the organisation.

It has been suggested that 'if implemented effectively, clinical audit would clearly reflect an improvement-based model of quality and be incorporated within the overall organisational strategy for quality improvement, encompassing collaboration between patients, carers, professionals and managers'[21]. Box 1.1 illustrates the key characteristics of clinical audit within the context of an improvement-based model.

Box 1.1 The characteristics of clinical audit within an improvement-based model (Harvey[21])

1. Level and scope of concern for quality
   Quality is made explicit in the form of agreed statements of best practice, for example, standards and guidelines. Responsibility for quality is vested in clinical teams involved in the care delivery process (including patients, carers and managers).

2. Definition of quality
   Quality is defined as the search for ways to continuously improve patient care and clinical audit is a mechanism by which this is achieved. In seeking improvement, there is a clear commitment to action, through closing the audit cycle and implementing changes in practice.

3. Control over the process of care delivery
   Clinical teams involved in care delivery are able to assume responsibility for planning, implementing, evaluating and taking action on care. This is reflected in decentralised work structures, with devolved decision-making and control. The manager plays a key role as a leader, in an enabling and supporting role.

4. Views of team members
   All team members are equally valued and respected, both from within the team and from outside. Methods of team working clearly encompass mutual trust and recognition.

5. Focus and means of achieving quality
   There is a central focus on improving the processes of care. Quality and audit form an integral part of everyday practice.

In order to sustain a programme of clinical audit it cannot be imposed. The involvement of the multi-professional clinical team must be nurtured by good training, facilitation and support from the wider organisation, factors that are discussed in Chapter 7. If practice is to change, clinical audit must be led by the clinical staff involved with the issue under review, in collaboration with managers, audit staff and patients.

 Redesign the audit cycle as a spiral showing how it might relate to clinical effectiveness and quality improvement.

Summary

- Clinical audit thrives in organisations where staff are valued.
- Clinical audit is about continuous improvement.
- Responsibility for clinical audit is devolved to clinical teams.

Having looked at a broad range of issues that affect clinical audit, the next four chapters examine the practicalities of an individual project and follow the path of the four phases of an audit cycle through defining best practice, implementation, measuring and taking action where necessary. The clinical audit cycle shown in Figure 1.2 sets out some of the detail these chapters address.

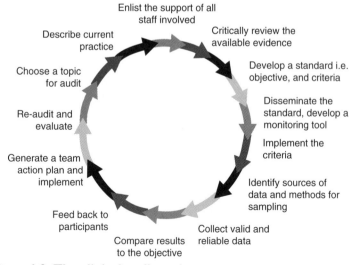

Figure 1.2 **The clinical audit cycle.**

References

1. Nightingale F 1872 Address from Miss Nightingale to the probationer Nurses in the 'Nightingale Fund' School, at St Thomas' Hospital and the Nurses who were formally trained there. Printed for private circulation, May 1872, p1
2. Pearson A 1987 Nursing quality measurement: quality assurance methods for peer review. Wiley, Chichester
3. Department of Health 1993 Clinical audit – meeting and improving standards in health care. DoH, London
4. Batstone G and Edwards M 1994 Clinical audit – how do we proceed? Southampton Medical Journal Jan 1994, 13–19
5. Mann T 1996 Clinical audit in the NHS. NHSE, Leeds
6. CRAG 1993 The interface between clinical audit and management. The Scottish Office, Edinburgh, p10
7. College of Speech and Language Therapists 1993 Audit: a workbook for speech and language therapists. CLST, London
8. Standing J 1985 Pressure Sore Survey: Somerset Health Authority. Somerset Health Authority: Taunton
9. Waterlow J 1991 A policy that protects. Professional Nurse Feb. 258–264
10. Hibbs P 1988 Action against pressure sores. Nursing Times 84 (13): 68–73
11. Collier M, Cole A 1997 Pressure area care: professional issues. Nursing Times 93(6): 9–12
12. Department of Health 1993 Pressure sores, a key quality indicator. HMSO, London
13. Department of Health 1997 The new NHS. Modern, dependable. HMSO, London
14. Department of Health 1998 A first class service: quality in the new NHS. HMSO, London
15. Royal College of Nursing 1998 Guidance for nurses on clinical governance. Royal College of Nursing, London
16. Morrell C, Harvey G, Kitson AL 1995 The reality of practitioner based quality improvement, report no. 14. National Institute for Nursing, Oxford
17. Ford P, Walsh M 1994 New rituals for old. Butterworth Heinemann, Oxford
18. Mallett J, Bailey C 1996 Manual of clinical nursing procedures. Blackwell, Oxford
19. Royal College of Nursing 1996 The RCN Clinical Effectiveness Initiative: a strategic framework. RCN, London, p3
20. Harvey G 1993 Which way to quality? National Institute for Nursing, Oxford
21. Harvey G 1996 Quality in health care: traditions, influences and future directions. International Journal for Quality in Health Care 8(4): 341–350

2

Defining best practice

This chapter covers:

- identifying an area for clinical audit
- describing current practice
- enlisting the support of all staff involved
- identifying a facilitator and a leader
- setting the ground rules for meetings
- critically reviewing the available evidence
- developing the standard
- formulating criteria
- refining criteria.

Identifying an area for clinical audit

Topic selection is critical and needs very careful thought and planning since significant resources are invested in any clinical audit project. The area identified must address important aspects of practice or concerns about quality of care. In the past nurses in particular have tried to write 'standards for everything', with the appearance of vast quality manuals which resemble what used to be called the procedure book[1]. It has been suggested that the aim of embarking upon an audit project is to 'release creativity and innovation'[2] and this requires careful thought in the selection of topics. Your reasons for choosing a topic might include those listed in Box 2.1

Box 2.1 Prioritising clinical audit topics

- A review of the patients' perspective on quality of care
- An area of high cost, volume or risk
- Evidence of a serious quality problem, e.g. patient complaints, infection rates
- The availability of systematic reviews of research or national clinical guidelines

> **Box 2.1 Prioritising clinical audit topics (*contd.*)**
> ■ Requests for data from a national audit project
> ■ Requirements of local commissioning groups or health
>   authorities
> ■ The possibility of sustainable improvement

To prioritise the topics being suggested by the team the above list could be used as the basis for a scoring system. Potential subjects for clinical audit are given a score between one and three for all of the factors listed. The highest scoring topic would then be selected for development into a clinical audit project.

 List some topics for clinical audit which you think would be appropriate for your clinical area. Develop a grid to include the factors above and score each topic accordingly to determine your priorities.

When choosing a topic for a clinical audit project it is worth checking whether someone else locally has already started work on the subject. Many organisations find it helpful to classify and index their clinical audit projects and to keep a record of projects in progress. In this way others are able to make sure that work is not repeated.

There are a number of ways in which projects can be indexed. Some organisations have used the headings *topic*, *sub-topic* and *client group* to classify projects, others use some form of code or key word. This is particularly useful if someone needs to see at a glance all projects pertinent to care of older adults, or infection control.

Most projects are developed for a specific clinical area, e.g. primary care or orthopaedics. Staff from other clinical areas may wish to address the same topic but for a different client group, so good indexing helps with the sharing of information to minimise repetition. On the example forms in Appendix 3 this classification is called 'reference' and can be used in any way that is considered useful locally.

Describing current practice

Once the focus of your project is decided it is worth taking stock and reflecting upon the state of practice before the clinical audit project gets underway. The purpose of collating data at this early stage is to describe current practice in a way that illustrates the problems and areas for improvement. In building up a good picture of current practice you can then see any improvement. By not collecting data at this stage there is a risk that improvement in practice may not be captured as experience suggests that much of the practice development happens as the criteria are implemented. The next chapter suggests collecting baseline data as soon as you have developed your monitoring tool. This will complement the information you collate at this early stage of the project.

There will be existing sources of information which can be brought together in order to provide an overview of the aspect of care under review. These could include:

- letters from patients, complaints or comments from external agencies
- critical incident reports – where members of staff have described and analysed important concerns following one incident
- summaries of team meetings or grand round where the issue has been discussed
- information from routine data sources including numbers of patients involved
- variance data from care pathways
- data collected from externally applied audits – educational audit, or national audit projects
- patient stories[3] or feedback from focus groups
- direct observation of care.

Enlisting the support of all those involved

At this planning stage it is vital to seek support from managers, the clinical audit committee, the clinical director and any others within the wider organisation and patients for whom the project has implications. The most effective way to enlist support is by forming a project group – the clinical audit group.

The clinical audit group should ideally comprise six to eight members. It is important that this group should be representative of all those who will be working with or affected by the project. This will include members of all the professional groups involved and, where possible, the recipients of the service, or representatives participating on their behalf.

For example, if the standard relates to supporting newly diagnosed diabetic children in the community, the team determining it may include a diabetic nurse specialist, general practitioner, school nurse, health visitor or district nurse, along with representatives of the diabetic child, such as the parents or members of a local support group.

These people are responsible for relaying information to and from their colleagues and thus the success of the project depends on their enthusiasm and ability to involve the wider team. Multi-professional teamwork is discussed again in Chapter 7.

At the first meeting it is worth identifying group members' experience of audit. This needs to be conducted in a relaxed atmosphere where people feel comfortable to be honest about their views on audit. It may be that some group members have no experience of audit and time for training needs to be identified. Alternatively, there may be colleagues who have considerable experience of audit and these skills can be utilised. Problems can sometimes arise when group members have very different experiences of clinical audit and these tensions need to be handled sensitively, valuing each individual's contribution.

You may find that professional colleagues have used different approaches or audit methods. This can lead to problems around defining terms. For example, confusion over the use of the term standard, by which one person means a percentage target and another means a statement of best practice, is enough to cause tension within a team. Team members need to be aware that they may be using terms differently and you need to come to some agreement about how they are to be defined for your particular project.

Identifying a facilitator and leader

The need for sensitivity and valuing of individual contributions can be lost if meetings are run as formal committees. Throughout its 12 year history of work in this area the RCN have advocated the need for someone working with the group who can take on an empowering and enabling role. This person is usually referred to as the *facilitator*. The facilitator is someone who has experience, both in the field of quality improvement, and of group dynamics. Their role is to support the group and guide the process of working through the clinical audit cycle.

The facilitator is often someone who is not immediately involved in the service being evaluated. This helps them to remain objective and to focus on the process of quality improvement, rather than the content of the subject area being addressed. There are a number of potential sources of facilitators. There may be people with facilitation skills in your organisation's clinical audit office or primary care audit group. It may also be worth contacting your local education providers. Within the nursing profession lecturers are expected to retain clinical links and involvement in a clinical audit project may be one useful way of doing this.

Training officers within human resource or personnel departments are another possible source of help, as are other staff within your organisation with a specific remit for practice development. In primary health care and in small organisations it may be more difficult to find help with facilitation. It may therefore be worth considering sending a member of your own team to train as a facilitator. The facilitator's role is discussed in more detail in Chapter 8.

In addition to the facilitator's role, it is useful to appoint a group leader from within the clinical team. This person's role is to act as the leader on a day-to-day basis. This involves taking responsibility for organising meetings, communicating with the group, receiving feedback and ensuring agreed actions are carried out.

Setting the ground rules for meetings

Having identified a group, with a named facilitator and leader, it is important that they should establish clear ground rules (Box 2.2). This includes clarifying roles and responsibilities within the group, and identifying other issues that are important to members. These might include the need to respect starting and finishing times of meetings and ensuring that problems are addressed openly.

Good planning is essential to effective meetings. The group need to have clear achievable goals or aims and objectives so that they can see that progress is being made. Agendas and minutes may help to structure the meetings, though some groups prefer a less formal approach. As a minimum, action agreed with names and target dates should be recorded.

Box 2.2　Creating ground rules

BLOOD TRANSFUSION AUDIT GROUP

The group meets at 1 p.m. on the third Thursday of each month. All meetings start on time and end one hour later.

Anyone unable to attend informs the group leader and sends a named alternate.

Group members are responsible for the flow of information to and from the people they represent.

The group leader is responsible for ensuring that the project meets with the Trust's Code of Good Practice for Clinical Audit.

The group facilitator is responsible for providing tea and coffee.

All group members are committed to the achievement of the aims and objectives.

Aims:

To coordinate the development of the blood transfusion process within the Trust.

To ensure clinical staff, managers and patients are kept informed of the project's progress.

Objectives:

To have Trust-wide standards ready for implementation within 6 months.

To audit practice across the Trust within 12 months.

To re-audit practice within 18 months.

To use existing communication channels to update all those affected by the project quarterly.

Reviewing the available evidence

The first task of the group is to critically appraise the available evidence for the topic concerned. We are using the term evidence to include the findings of research, professional expertise and the preferences of service users. Research evidence is available from a number of sources. As well as searching the indexes in your local library a number of national databases exist, the details of which can be found in Appendix 2. National clinical guidelines may exist for the practice issue you are addressing, in which case the task of the group is to appraise them and adapt them for local use.

Sometimes no research has been done on a clinical area chosen as the topic for audit. This might affect your decision to continue, as the amount of available evidence is one important consideration in choosing a topic. If you make the decision to proceed in the absence of research, because the area is a priority in all the other ways listed in Box 2.1, then you will need to consider other types of evidence; professional consensus and patient preferences.

Using the findings of research

Information located during a search for evidence must be critically appraised to make sure it is of a sufficient quality and current enough to be valid and reliable as a basis for practice. The findings of randomised controlled trials (RCTs), observational and experimental research can provide evidence of effectiveness, and critical appraisal must ensure that the research itself is well designed.

Obviously the more research that exists, the better able you will be to make informed decisions about effective practice. The problem this poses is the time and effort necessary to locate and appraise all the information. Increasingly, systematic reviews exist which have been constructed so that the evidence has already been located and appraised. Criteria for appraising research papers and systematic reviews are available from the Critical Appraisal Skills Programme (see Appendix 2).

Using clinical guidelines

As you search for evidence you may find national clinical guidelines available for the clinical audit topic you have chosen. These clinical guidelines could be presented in a format where the recommendations lend themselves to use as standards, either by forming statements of objectives or by incorporation as criteria. Guidelines need careful adaptation for use locally so as not to undermine the research evidence on which they are based. This process of local adaptation is discussed more fully in Chapter 9 in the section on guidelines. Factors you will need to consider in the local interpretation of any nationally or externally developed guideline include:

- Is it achievable in your workplace?
- Is it achievable for the clients you work with?
- What needs to change to make it achievable?
- Are there options given for adaptation?
- Are the recommendations desirable for the clients and staff you work with?

An instrument has been produced by a team led from St George's Hospital Medical School[4] to assist practitioners in the process of guideline appraisal.

Using professional expertise

In the absence of research, there may be a current and accepted consensus of opinion based on the consideration of a multi-professional panel of experts in the field. There may also be consensus of opinion published in the form of guidelines from self-help or support groups, which explicitly include the opinions and preferences of the user group they represent.

Where there is no published expert consensus, best practice will have to be agreed upon by a process of professional consensus locally. This process may be extremely time-consuming as it involves ensuring that all the relevant groups are thoroughly consulted.

Incorporating the preferences of service users

Whether or not there are other sorts of evidence it is important to include the views of the recipients of the service in determining best practice locally. This can be done in a number of ways such as contacting local support groups concerned with the clinical issue under review, using focus groups, interviews or patient stories[3]. These techniques for involving service users are discussed more fully in Chapter 7.

Learning from the experiences of others involved in clinical audit

It is worth finding out whether there are good quality audit projects from colleagues who have considered the topic in the past and are further round the cycle. It is often helpful to see how others have decided upon best practice and also to look at the tools and techniques they have used to monitor and develop their practice. Increasingly, national clinical audit projects are being developed (see Chapter 6). It may be worth checking whether such a project exists for the practice issue you are addressing.

Figure 2.1 suggests a route to search for evidence, along with some potential sources. It is expected that many of these data sources will be brought together by the National Institute for Clinical Excellence, described in the White Paper 'The New NHS'[5].

1. Are systematic reviews of the evidence available?

Sources include:

Royal Colleges and Professional Organisations

The NHS Centre for Reviews and Dissemination (including database called DARE – database of abstracts of reviews of effectiveness, available on the internet, floppy disk and CD Rom). Items on this database are critically appraised. NHSCRD also produce regular systematic reviews of the evidence in the form of publications called Effectiveness Matters and Effective Health Care Bulletins.

The UK Cochrane Centre is an organisation which conducts rigorous systematic reviews in a variety of areas. They have a database which is available on CD-Rom and floppy disk. There is also a separate database dedicated specifically to midwifery and childbirth. Items on the Cochrane database are critically appraised.

Journals and newsletters specifically dedicated to publishing systematic reviews include Evidence–Based Medicine, Evidence–Based Nursing, Journal of Clinical Effectiveness.

Health Care Technology Assessments have been commissioned by the Health Service Executive and some involve systematic reviews in a variety of areas.

↓

2. Are there any individual research projects?

Sources include:

Journal articles – to find relevant articles try using index and abstracts in the library or the libraries' own in-house databases. Libraries generally offer access to other databases such as Cochrane. Royal Colleges, professional organisations, academic institutions, independent research organisations – all carry out individual pieces of research.

Libraries and information sources which specialise in specific clinical areas – use an information directory to locate the appropriate ones.

Clinical databases such as MEDLINE and Cinahl (Cumulative Index to Nursing and Allied Health Literature) collect together articles from a very large number of clinical and medical journals and they can be searched at most clinical libraries (items are not critically appraised). Health plan database has health care management articles.

↓

(cont'd)

3. Are national clinical guidelines available?
Sources include:
Royal Colleges and professional organisations
Self-help and service user support agencies
Agency for Health Care Policy and Research (USA)
Health Care Evaluation Unit, St George's Hospital, London
Scottish Intercollegiate Guidelines Network

↓

4. Are Audit and Quality Projects available?
Sources include:
Royal Colleges and professional organisations
Some specialist Audit Information Sources, e.g. National Co-ordinating Unit for Clinical Audit in Family Planning, Nursing and Midwifery Audit Information Service.
National and Regional Audit services; National Centre for Clinical Audit, Eli Lilly National Clinical Audit Centre, Clinical Audit Association, regional audit resources, e.g. Lothian Audit. Patient involvement issues from the College of Health.

Figure 2.1 Sources of evidence.

For an audit topic you have chosen use the flow diagram in Figure 2.1 to design a search strategy, setting out where you will look for your evidence.

Developing the standard

Having reviewed the literature and assimilated the evidence, the next step involves setting a standard. A standard needs to set out what is best practice and give some indication of how that is to be achieved. Before describing this in detail it is worth clarifying the way in which the term standard is used.

The terms standard and criterion have been used differently by different authors and the various professional groups across health care. There has been much confusion over the use of these terms in recent years. Nurses have generally used the term standard as defined in the top left section of Box 2.3, with standard setting representing the development of statements of best practice. Medical audit has understood standards, as described in the bottom left section, in terms of expected compliance rates usually expressed as a percentage.

Box 2.3 Definitions

Standard	**Criterion**
A statement which outlines an objective with guidance for its achievement given in the form of criteria sets which specify required resources, activities and predicted outcomes[6].	An item or variable which enables the achievement of a standard (broad objective of care) and the evaluation of whether it has been achieved or not[6].
A standard describes the level of care to be achieved for any particular criterion[7].	The term is used to describe a definable and measurable item of health care which describes quality, and which can be used to assess it[7].

To be consistent with the approach that the RCN has taken for many years, whilst recognising the confusion that has occurred, standard is taken to mean the definition of best practice which may be expressed in terms of an objective and criteria.

Objective – a broad statement of good practice based on the best possible evidence

Criterion – an item necessary to the achievement of best practice

A standard is developed in the form of objectives and criteria. Criteria provide the more detailed and practical information on how to achieve the objective. Thus, the objective sets out best practice, and the criteria indicate how that is to be achieved.

An example of an objective is:

Objective: Every infant has access to immunisation against diphtheria, tetanus, pertussis, polio and influenza (B) before they are 6 months old.

Formulating criteria

While the objective gives a broad indication of good practice, it does not provide much detail about how you reach this. This is the role of the *criteria*. These refer to the resources (structure) which you need, the actions (process) that must be undertaken, and the results (outcomes) you intend to achieve.

Structure criteria (what you need) refer to resources in the system that are necessary for the successful achievement of the objective under review. This may include a consideration of staffing levels and skill mix, requirements for knowledge and expertise, organisational arrangements, and the provision of equipment and physical space.

Process criteria (what you do) refer to actions and decisions undertaken by staff, in conjunction with clients, in order to achieve the specified objective. These actions may include assessment, education, evaluation and documentation. Process criteria may refer to existing policies, procedures or protocols.

Outcome criteria (what you expect) describe the desired results of the project from the perspective of the recipient of the service. Outcomes are typically expressed in terms such as physical or behavioural response to an intervention, reported health status, and level of knowledge and satisfaction.

Some teams choose not to classify their criteria as structure, process and outcome, preferring instead to use unclassified lists of criteria or indicators. The advantage of separating the criteria in this way is that if an outcome is not achieved the structures and processes necessary have already been identified and so the source of the problem should be obvious. Audit of just outcome could mean that there is insufficient information to develop an action plan for improvement.

You may find it helpful to adapt one of the forms in Appendix 3 to help the group identify the structure, process and outcome criteria for the objective they have identified. These are derived using the information collected in your search for evidence. You may also wish to consider:

- beliefs and values about the practice issue held by team members
- acceptability to patients/clients or user groups
- existing policies, procedures and protocols
- relevant strategies, initiatives and systems within the organisation.

When identifying criteria it is not expected that you will identify an outcome and a process for every structure criterion as this
is unnecessarily repetitive. There are times when it is difficult to
determine which area a particular criterion most naturally fits[8],
but with experience this becomes significantly easier.

It is also important to make sure that outcomes are not mere-
ly processes stated in the past tense. Outcomes are the antici-
pated results of implementing structure and process criteria
usually expressed in terms of patient behaviour, knowledge or
signs of recovery. It may be useful to ask yourselves 'what do
you expect the patient to be able to do now that they could not
do before the intervention of the health care team?'

Preoperative fasting example

Eilish Toal, The Royal Hospitals, Belfast

This project came out of a concern that patients were arriving in theatres
following extended periods of preoperative fasting. The project began by
trying to ascertain existing hospital policy and collecting data to examine
current practice – seeing how long patients were actually fasting. In addition nurses' existing knowledge levels were evaluated about the dangers
to the patient who is exposed to a prolonged preoperative fast.

Having described current practice in this way, a standard was set for
preoperative fasting by a multi-professional group drawing on the best
available research evidence.

Preoperative fasting standard

Objective: All adult patients are fasted preoperatively in accordance
with research-based evidence.

Structure	Process	Outcome
Research evidence is available at ward level.	Care is carried out according to the protocol agreed by all professions.	Prolonged fasting of patients preopera-tively is minimised.
Staff are aware of the standard and its rationale.	In exceptional cir-cumstances where longer fasting occurs appropriate mouth care is offered.	Hospital practice on preoperative fasting is reviewed regularly.

Refining criteria

Having formulated an objective it is very easy to find suddenly that the group has identified huge lists of criteria necessary for the implementation of the objective. It is then important to pare the list down to its necessary components. This can be done by applying the mnemonic DREAM, and asking the question *is this criterion*:

- Distinct – does it identify something new, not repeating other criteria?
- Relevant – is it crucial to the achievement of the objective?
- Evidence-based – is the source of information clear?
- Achievable – is it realistic within current resources?
- Measurable – most importantly, can it be measured?

These discussions may cause some debate within the team. As a rule it is worth keeping your criteria as succinct as possible. This may mean referring to other documents that will then need creating. For example, your process criteria may list actions to be carried out by a staff member. It might then be appropriate to make reference to policies, procedures or protocols. When such documents do not already exist you may wish to develop a local guideline or protocol as in the example below.

Using an audit project that already exists within your organisation, apply the DREAM mnemonic to the criteria and see how you can refine them.

In this example much of the work of the defining phase of the leg ulcer project has gone into the development of a protocol for assessment and treatment. The group have chosen to set an objective and the criteria needed to achieve the objective are described within the protocol.

The defining phase: an example

Chrissy Dunn, Senior Nurse, Practice Development

As a part of the King's Fund PACE Programme, the Royal Berkshire and Battle Hospitals NHS Trust in conjunction with West Berkshire

Priority Care Service have developed a project looking at the treatment of venous leg ulcers in the area.

For a long time there has been a Tissue Viability Group in West Berkshire with representation from a wide range of clinical and managerial staff from hospital and community bases, and from Berkshire health authority. This group had identified a lack of consistency in treatment across the community. In addition, it had recently become apparent that when people came into hospital with leg ulcers, the ward nurses did not know how to continue the treatment prescribed in the community.

Using the criteria in Box 2.1 this was clearly a priority topic for clinical audit because:

- the inappropriate treatment of venous leg ulcers was causing unnecessary pain and suffering to patients
- the total cost to the NHS of leg ulcers has been estimated at between £300 million and £600 million per annum
- there has been considerable work done in developing the evidence base for the treatment of venous leg ulcers including a systematic review[9] and a national clinical guideline[10]
- the tissue viability group felt that the possibility of sustainable improvement was within their remit and
- a national initiative (the PACE Programme) had given the group the motivation and resources to embark upon it.

The Tissue Viability Group agreed a project plan and set up four working groups. A group was convened to see through the defining phase and develop an assessment tool and protocol.

Objective: There is consistent, evidence-based assessment and treatment of leg ulcers across community and hospital settings in accordance with an agreed assessment and treatment protocol.

The assessment and protocol working group included a ward sister, a practice nurse, an infection control nurse, a pharmacist, a dermatologist and a GP. I am the project leader and when necessary the group facilitator, as I have many years of experience in facilitating clinical audit groups. This group met only three times as most of the work was done outside the meetings by phone and fax.

The group set out a search strategy and searched the published literature for evidence of leg ulcer treatments. A systematic review has since been published[9]. We also wrote to the academic departments around the UK where we knew that current research was underway.

The content of our document was reasonably easy to sort out as there was strong research evidence. More time was spent agreeing the style of the document – ward nurses wanted something to go into patients' notes and district nurses wished to be able to carry it in their pocket. Small groups were circulated with countless drafts and we were very pleased to have produced the final version in 18 months.

The protocol has now been implemented across West Berkshire. We calculated at the beginning of the audit project that the average cost per person per week of treating a venous leg ulcer was £99; after three months of graduated compression bandaging this had been reduced to £42.

The cycle does not finish here, defining best practice is only the beginning! The next stage is to implement the objectives and criteria before monitoring their effect.

Summary

- The first step in achieving quality improvement is the defining phase, which involves selecting an area of care that is a source of concern or has arisen from new organisational or care developments.
- The rationale for developing a standard on the topic area chosen should be made explicit and a representative group convened.
- The evidence on which to base the standard can be derived from several sources including research, professional experience, existing policies and procedures and patients' views.
- Standards can be presented as *objectives* which describe the broad outcomes for care and *criteria sets* which specify the resources (structure) and activities (process) required to achieve the objective and the expected results (outcomes).
- Criteria are refined by asking whether they are distinct, relevant, evidence-based, achievable and measurable.

References

1. Shelley H 1992 Mission impossible? Nursing Times 88: 16, 37
2. Ford P, Walsh M 1994 New rituals for old. Butterworth Heinemann, Oxford
3. Adair L 1994 The patient's agenda. Nursing Standard 9(9): 20–23
4. Cluzeau F, Littlejohns P, Grimshaw J, Feder G 1997 Appraisal instrument for clinical guidelines. HCEU, St George's Hospital Medical School, London
5. Department of Health 1997 The new NHS. Modern, dependable. The Stationery Office, London
6. Royal College of Nursing 1990 Quality patient care – the Dynamic Standard Setting System. Scutari, Harrow
7. Irvine D, Irvine S 1991 Making sense of audit. Radcliffe Medical Press, Oxford
8. Girvin J 1995 Standard setting – a practical approach. Macmillan, London
9. Fletcher A, Cullum N, Sheldon TA 1997 A systematic review of compression for venous leg ulcers. BMJ 315: 576
10. RCN Institute, Centre for Evidence Based Nursing, School of Nursing, Midwifery and Health Visiting, University of Manchester 1998 Clinical practice guidelines: the management of patients with venous leg ulcers. RCN, London

3

Implementing best practice and preparing to monitor

This chapter covers:

- preparing to monitor
- disseminating and implementing the standard
- obtaining agreement for the standard
- setting target dates for implementation and audit.

Preparing to monitor

Before implementing your standard it is worth considering how you will measure the effect of this process. Developing your criteria into an audit tool at this stage will help further refine the content and this will allow for the collection of data as a baseline before the systematic implementation and the consequent changes in practice. There are three elements to consider in preparing for implementation: *developing a measurement tool, validity and reliability, and collecting baseline data.*

Developing a measurement tool

Having refined your criteria once already, the emphasis is now on whether the criteria are measurable. Structure criteria can usually be listed – they either exist or do not. Process criteria may be observable either directly or by assessing the result, e.g. it may not be necessary to watch staff completing a multi-professional discharge plan, since it is possible to check whether it has been completed at an appropriate time. Outcomes are usually stated in terms of patient knowledge or behaviours. It may then be necessary to ask patients about their experience of care, or whether they can demonstrate a skill they have been taught.

Where research has established an attributable relationship between an intervention and an outcome it is particularly appropriate to focus on measuring the intervention, i.e. process.

If there is no proven link between process and outcome it is wise to measure both.

If you are using clinical guidelines as the basis for your criteria there may well be an audit tool formulated with the guidelines for you to use. Often there are audit pointers, highlighting areas for monitoring. There are also a number of measurement tools and patient satisfaction questionnaires which have been designed for research studies and may be useful for clinical audit on the same topic[1]. It has been suggested that the choice of whether to use a particular measure should be made against a number of key criteria[2]:

- reliability and validity
- responsiveness (or sensitivity) to change
- clinical utility
- feasibility of data collection.

Developing measurement tools is a skilled task and it may be helpful to call on the expertise of clinical audit staff within your organisation or others locally who have experience in this area. This is one aspect of the audit process which draws heavily on the skills used in research. This can sometimes lead to confusion about the differences between research and audit. Although the purpose of audit is different, the design of a project needs to be considered with a similar thoroughness. You will find a number of research texts which describe in detail the issues highlighted here in Appendix 6.

Some of the common formats for data collection tools are described below.

Checklists are particularly useful for structure criteria, for reviewing patient records, or direct observation of care. The criteria must be very clearly stated so that they are not open to interpretation. For example, 'a thorough assessment is recorded on admission to the ward': one person's view of what constitutes a thorough assessment might be quite different from another person's. It is therefore important to be specific and perhaps refer to local policies, procedures or protocols. It is also useful to allow space for comments on any checklist as this enables reasons for non-compliance to be recorded.

The disadvantage of using checklists for record review is that the assessment can only be as good as the records themselves, which is fine if the project is about good record keeping. It is important not to rely on records alone to describe the quality of patient care as they may not provide an accurate picture.

Questionnaires can provide a good method for obtaining feedback from patients. Questions must be carefully formulated to ensure that they do not direct the replies, and it is worth bearing in mind that response rates from postal questionnaires are commonly low. There are a number of ways to structure a questionnaire[3] including the use of answer boxes, scales and space for free response. An example of answer boxes might be:

Did staff respect your privacy and confidentiality?
☐ Yes   ☐ No

Answering 'yes' suggests that privacy and confidentiality were respected all the time, answering 'no' implies the opposite. There is no means of answering in a way which reflects the perception that staff respected privacy and confidentiality some of the time or that staff respected privacy but the ward layout meant that confidentiality was very difficult to maintain. A better approach might be:

Did you feel that staff respected your privacy?

☐   ☐   ☐   ☐
all the time   most of the time   some of the time   never

Did you feel that staff respected your confidentiality?

☐   ☐   ☐   ☐
all the time   most of the time   some of the time   never

Please add your comments:

Interviews can give service users the opportunity to provide detailed descriptive feedback to staff. They can also allow the interviewer to ensure that the question has been understood. However, patients or their carers may find it difficult to express critical views and the skill of the interviewer may influence the outcome. Interviews can be structured, semi-structured or unstructured depending on the nature of the information required[4].

Data can be tape recorded and transcribed either in full or selectively, or notes can be made by the interviewer or observer. To ensure that views are represented accurately it can be useful to ask the person concerned to read the summary and say whether it is a true account of what they said.

Observation of care is useful to identify what people actually do. Normally a written record of observation is made, though video recordings are increasingly used. Within a climate of trust, openness and learning, observation can be a very useful tool for giving clinical staff feedback on their practice. It may be sufficient to record observational data on a structured checklist. However, it could be valuable to the team to write a fuller account of what is happening, including personal reflections on any interactions between staff and patients[5].

There is debate in the research literature about the extent to which the observer should be a part of the environment concerned. This can be seen as a continuum from complete participant to complete observer[6], and decisions need to be taken about who is appropriate for the project. In order to achieve a balance between objectivity and understanding of the particular situation, it may be helpful for a team member to observe practice with someone from outside the team and to feed this information back to practitioners, reflecting on their different interpretations and perspectives.

There is no method suitable for all situations and the right approach needs to be chosen for the particular project. A combination of methods is often needed to address the various criteria.

Validity and reliability

Validity and reliability are important concepts in the design of measurement tools. Every audit criterion or question is measuring a particular variable and we need to assess how good it is at its job, i.e. how reliable it is and how valid.

If the measure is used over and over again it should give you the same results; this is *reliability*, sometimes assessed in terms of stability and consistency. As a part of your pilot project it may be useful for two people to use your measurement tool simultaneously to see if they get the same results, this would be testing for inter-rater reliability. If you are using a questionnaire you could ask patients to fill it in once and then again to see if you get the same responses to assess stability or divide the questionnaire into two asking the same questions twice in slightly different ways and comparing the results to assess consistency.

Validity describes whether the criteria are measuring what they are supposed to. Using a questionnaire, you will need to consider whether the questions are understandable and unambiguous, as described above. With observation or interviewing the validity of data may be affected by the person collecting it. Training and supervision for that individual may be necessary. Again this highlights the importance of piloting data collection methods.

It is important to try out your tools before the main data collection phase. In this way problem areas are highlighted and can be rectified. Commonly people find ambiguities in the wording of questions at this stage.

For a measurement tool already in use in your organisation, consider its reliability and validity and how it could be improved.

Collecting baseline data

It may be useful to use this opportunity to collect 'baseline' data, providing a starting point from which progress can be measured. Right at the beginning of the project you will have described current practice in a variety of ways using whatever evidence was available. This is a good opportunity to collect more structured data before your criteria are implemented. At the same time it is worth recognising that the project may already have raised awareness of the issue under review and influenced practice to some extent.

For consistency the sample size for your baseline data collection should be the same as that used later in the project but this depends on the nature of the project, the ease with which data can be collected and the extent to which it is dependent on clinical staff whose agreement may not have been sought at this stage. Realistically you need to collect data as widely as is practical given that much of the project planning remains to be done. The purpose of clinical audit is not to give a definitive view of changing practice, but an indicator of the quality of practice. Given the importance of involving staff the data is bound to be coloured by their awareness of the project so this needs to be carefully considered as the timing of data collection is planned.

This chapter sets out a series of sequential steps. In reality implementation and preparing for measurement need to occur in parallel. Taking into account the principle of involvement and the ethical issue of consent (see Chapter 7) you may decide that it is not appropriate to collect data until all staff have been informed of the project and given the opportunity to comment. Having disseminated the standard and obtained support, it would then be appropriate to collect baseline data as the first action on the implementation plan before changes in practice are introduced.

Implementing the standard

Once the objective has been agreed, the criteria refined and a measuring tool developed, the focus moves to implementing the standard. Getting the implementation right is essential to the success and adoption of good practice in your area. This stage involves three important steps:

- letting the wider team know about the project
- obtaining agreement to proceed with implementation and
- agreeing realistic target dates for implementation and audit.

Disseminating the standard

Throughout the process of writing your objective and compiling criteria, you should be taking steps to inform and involve all those who will be affected. In other words, the sense of ownership must be shared as widely as possible and should not simply rest with the clinical audit group. Promoting a sense of ownership involves setting up feedback systems to give information to colleagues and provide them with an opportunity to comment. These might include:

- circulation of draft documents
- notice boards
- newsletters
- hand-over meetings
- other regular meetings
- ward rounds.

This type of information exchange is especially important around the time of implementation. If staff feel that they have not had the opportunity to comment on the practices described, they are unlikely to implement them.

Obtaining agreement from the wider team

Following dissemination, the clinical audit group must obtain more formal recognition by seeking the support of senior staff within the organisation; this may be the clinical audit committee or quality steering group. It could also be the clinical director or manager – whoever is ultimately responsible for the resources involved in implementation. However, it is important that this process is seen as one of supporting the project, rather than as a mechanism for 'marking' or vetting. It is worth remembering that clinical audit projects often have implications for clinical units across and beyond the organisation and getting agreement may involve an extensive process of consultation. This relates back to the need to ensure that the necessary communication channels and support are in place when negotiating the selection of topics for clinical audit.

Setting target dates for implementation and audit

One of the assumptions the group cannot afford to make is that simply as a result of setting out a new document, practice will change. In planning for implementation, the group needs to consider what changes need to take place before the criteria can be implemented in practice, who is responsible for these changes and how long they will take. This involves working through the structure and process criteria identifying those which do not currently exist and the time needed to implement them. For example:

Short term (<6 weeks) – in order to meet a standard on information for patients and visitors one of the structure criteria involves a board displaying photographs of all the staff; the implementation plan would include having the photographs taken and making up the display board.

Medium term (<6 months) – in a standard on day surgery the structure criteria may include information leaflets available for patients. Part of the implementation plan may therefore involve their development if they do not already exist.

Long term (> 6 months) – in a standard on care of intra-venous cannulae the criteria state that all relevant health care staff receive training in siting and maintaining a patent cannula. The implementation plan would include arranging appropriate training to fit in with the working patterns of all the staff concerned and ensuring that ongoing educational opportunities exist for new staff.

The group need to set themselves a realistic date by which they expect implementation to be complete. As well as agreeing the date for implementation, the group also set themselves a date to begin auditing or assessing their level of achievement. This date should fall some time after the agreed implementation date, allowing time for the innovations to become established in practice.

The group may decide to stage their implementation plan as in the following example.

From the example on preoperative fasting in Chapter 2, The Royal Hospitals, Belfast

A standard was set whose objective read: All adult patients are fasted preoperatively in accordance with research-based evidence. The baseline data collected in October 1996 described a situation where less than 3% of patients were fasting preoperatively in accordance with the research findings. Given the scale of the task in implementing best practice the team decided to stage their implementation by setting what was felt to be a more achievable goal. Therefore the team decided that by October 1997, 75% of patients would be fasted preoperatively for no longer than 6 hours for solids and 4 hours for fluids.

This second example describes the lessons learned from a previous attempt to implement the same standard and illustrates the development and use of local guidelines as a complementary part of the implementation phase.

The implementation of the Edinburgh Postnatal Depression Scale as part of a project within the Oxfordshire Community NHS Trust

Mary McClarey, Senior Nurse (1984–1995)

In Oxford in 1994, there was no agreement within the primary health care teams as to how postnatal depression should be recognised and treated. The health visitors felt the need to standardise the method of identification to enable them to measure the prevalence of postnatal depression and the GPs were concerned about the increasing number of new mothers coming to surgeries who were depressed.

Unsuccessful implementation

An earlier attempt by health visitors to introduce the use of the Edinburgh Postnatal Depression Scale[7-9] (EPDS) into their practice had failed, and two years later the problem of lack of consensus regarding the management of postnatal depression was still causing concern to midwives and health visitors. Having identified a lack of collaboration as one of the main barriers to implementing the change on that occasion, a second attempt was made, taking a more structured approach.

In the first attempt the health visitor team did not discuss the proposed change in practice with any other health professionals – GPs, the mental health unit and the midwifery service were all thought to have little to do with the proposed new practice. There was a diversity of practices developing between primary health care teams. In some teams health visitors were strongly discouraged by the GPs, who described the EPDS as a diagnostic tool and therefore encroaching on the doctor's role. They also expressed concern that their patients might be having therapy without the GP's knowledge.

This non-consultative approach did much to damage the cooperation within the teams as some health visitors, anxious not to confront the GPs but convinced that they should continue to use the EPDS, did so, concealing their actions from the other primary health care team members.

A second attempt

A multi-professional group, consisting of representatives of every health profession involved in providing care to women in the antenatal and postnatal period was set up. The group also included patient representation, voluntary organisations which gave support to families, and a commissioning health professional.

There were three main aims for the project:

- to improve detection rates and minimise the effects of postnatal depression by screening women using EPDS and coordinating therapy between professionals
- to train health visitors to use their skills more effectively with this group of women and to offer non-directive counselling where appropriate
- to raise the profile of postnatal depression for the benefit of patients and professionals.

Consultation

The clinical audit group met monthly to agree a strategy and began with a consultative process. The first step was to circulate a discussion paper to primary health care teams. This paper contained information on the rationale behind the proposed strategy, and aimed to elicit the teams' views about the project. The paper also contained a questionnaire to identify current practice and existing prevalence of postnatal depression and give the team members the opportunity to comment on the proposed new practice.

Awareness raising

The next stage was a meeting of all primary health care team members, with an extended invitation to staff involved in maternity and psychiatric services. This gave everyone an opportunity to share the results of the questionnaires, to update knowledge of postnatal depression and to seek options for a flexible and acceptable approach.

> **Objective:** all women in Oxfordshire are offered screening for postnatal depression twice within 8 months of childbirth, and action is taken accordingly.

Structure	Process	Outcome
Training and supervision are available for health visitors involved with screening for postnatal depression.	Postnatal depression is discussed with women by midwives in the antenatal period (at approx 36 weeks).	Screening for postnatal depression is offered to all women in a way that is acceptable to them.

Local guidelines exist for treatment of high scoring women.	6–8 weeks postnatal Offer EPDS and check score. Offer treatment according to local guideline. 6–8 months postnatal (as above)	The incidence of post natal depression is known. The incidence of severe postnatal depression is minimised by early detection.[10–12]

Implementation – the development of local guidelines

In order to keep the recommendations and the research-based evidence readily available, a document for inclusion in Oxfordshire's 'Guidelines for shared care' was drawn up. This acknowledges the health visitor input, keeps the GPs informed of the process and clarifies the referral criteria agreed between themselves and the psychiatric services. It also describes the options for drug dosages and gives information on the effect of medication on lactation and sleep patterns. The health authority press officer then became involved ensuring maximum publicity for new developments. Once agreed, the postnatal depression standard was launched using local press, television and radio.

Implementation – training and supervision

Local workshops for primary health care teams were developed outlining the change in practice and focusing on the evidence base underpinning this change. Every primary health care team had access to a health visitor who had been trained in non-directive counselling. Supervision by a clinical psychologist for those delivering the counselling had been negotiated and a referral route to psychiatric services from primary health care team members had been agreed. Midwives and psychologists had worked together to develop a sensitive format for antenatal discussions.

The next stage

One year after the implementation of the new practice the results of an audit demonstrated that the desired change in practice had occurred and that it had identified the incidence and reduced the morbidity of postnatal depression. An audit was also carried out on both the views of the patients on the acceptability of the treatment and of the health visitors' views on the practice of non-directive counselling. The results of this audit were shared at an open meeting, to which all primary health care team members were invited.

Participants were asked how they felt the strategy had influenced their working practice. They reported that having external support provided by the training and supervision had given health visitors and GPs a structure within which they could feel confident of the way they were working. Overall the multi-professional approach to this programme of care had improved communication within the team, had improved understanding of other health professionals' roles and had increased primary health care team cooperation within a wider context.

As an implementation strategy, identifying barriers to change and addressing them through a process of consultation and collaboration was successful. However, primary health care teams are ever changing and there will remain an ongoing training and consultation requirement to consolidate this new practice.

 Draw up an action plan to implement criteria you have developed to include how you will enlist the support of all those affected by the project.

Summary

- A measurement tool is developed from key elements of the standard.
- The measurement tool is tried out in practice to ensure it can be easily used.
- Baseline data are collected for comparison with practice after implementation of the standard.
- The clinical audit group should disseminate the information to all relevant staff and obtain agreement to enable the standard to be recognised and accepted.
- Once the criteria have been refined the group need to decide what changes need to take place, who is responsible for these changes and how long they will take.
- Target dates for implementation and audit should be set.

References

1. Bowling A 1995 Measuring disease: a review of disease specific quality of life measurement scales. Open University Press, Buckingham
2. Long A 1996 Exploring outcomes within audit. Outcomes Briefing 7: 15–19
3. Oppenheim AN 1992 Questionnaire design, interviewing and attitude measurement. Pinter, London
4. Rubin H, Rubin I 1995 Qualitative interviewing – the art of hearing data. Sage Publications, Thousand Oaks, California.
5. Polit D, Hungler B 1995 Nursing research, principles and methods, 3rd edn. Lippincott, Philadelphia
6. Hammersley M, Atkinson P 1995 Ethnography, 2nd edn. Routledge, New York
7. Cox J, Connor Y, Kendall R 1982 A prospective study of the psychiatric disorders of childbirth. British Journal of Psychiatry 140: 111–117.
8. Cox JL, Holden JM, Sagovsky R 1987 Detection of postnatal depression: development of a ten item Edinburgh postnatal depression scale. British Journal of Psychiatry 150: 782–786
9. Harris B, Huckle P, Johns S et al 1989 The use of rating scales to identify postnatal depression. British Journal of Psychiatry 154: 817
10. Cooper PJ, Campbell EA, Day A et al 1988 Non psychotic psychiatric disorder after childbirth: a prospective study of prevalence, incidence, course and nature. British Journal of Psychiatry 152: 799–804
11. Cullinan R 1991 Health visitor intervention in postnatal depression. Health Visitor 64(12): 412–414
12. Holden JM, Sagovsky R, Cox JL 1989 Counselling in a general practice setting: controlled study of health visitor intervention in treatment of postnatal depression. British Medical Journal 298: 223–226

4

Monitoring your achievement

This chapter covers:

- the importance of good measurement
- sources of audit data
- agreeing a sample and time-frame
- who should collect data
- staff and patient consent
- recording audit data
- comparison and analysis.

The importance of good measurement

There has been some controversy in the literature about what constitutes rigorous audit. It is felt that in the past staff have collected inadequate data because a project was considered *only* audit and therefore did not need to be conducted with the same rigour as research. It has been argued that audit is a form of clinical science[1] and should therefore be carried out with the same degree of rigour as research.

> There seems to be a general belief that we don't need skills in handling numbers beyond those gained at most primary schools: counting, percentages and decimals. Certainly there does not seem to be any widespread awareness of a need to be able to view figures with the sophistication required to extract the maximum information from them and avoid misleading conclusions. But why? Because it's only audit?[2]

This need for rigour must be held in tension with the relational aspects of the clinical audit process. It could be argued that an over emphasis on rigour risks alienating the very people whose confidence and skills are most likely to benefit from involvement in clinical audit. Planning the methods of data collection and analysis provides an opportunity to draw on the expertise of the team. It may be that there is a member of the project group who is highly numerate and another who has experience of qualitative data analysis. Your local clinical audit office may well be able to help at this stage. It is better to ask for help than to compromise the potential benefits to patient care.

Sources of audit data

As described in the previous section on developing an audit tool there are several obvious sources of data, including question-naires to or interviews with patients themselves, direct observa-tion of care and so on, where data are collected specifically for the clinical audit project. It is, however, worth considering the many pre-existing data sources collected routinely in the course of the health care process.

Patient records kept as a routine part of care are the obvious pre-existing data source. Hospital and general practice infor-mation systems store a wealth of data – patient administration, case-mix management, personnel, finance. Many of these data sources could have readily accessible information which, if applicable, would save time and effort if utilised. These data sources are particularly useful when looking for incidence of a particular problem. For example, a clinical audit project look-ing at health education of children with asthma in schools might find it useful to know the numbers of children admitted to their local hospital with acute asthma to compare with the national data.

In addition, 'research' fields on these established information systems can be used to collect specific information for audit. Other routinely collected data sources include:

- cancer registries
- infection control data
- discharge data
- contracts monitoring.

Agreeing a sample

The entire set of people to whom your project applies is called the *target population*. It may be that your project applies to a small population, for example children in sickle cell crisis, in which case it may be straightforward to collect data from the entire population. If the clinical audit topic is discharge from hospital, then you could have a very large population and collecting data from them all would be a huge undertaking. Sampling allows us to generalise on the basis of responses from a smaller group of the population concerned, in the hope that they are representative of the population as a whole. This smaller group or subset is a *sample*.

The purpose of the audit is to describe accurately the behaviour, thoughts or opinions of the whole population on the basis of data collected from a smaller sample. Opinion polls constantly strive to select samples which are representative of the population at large. The 1992 General Election was predicted to be a clear Labour victory according to the opinion polls. Their sampling procedures had led to a biased result which was evidently not representative of the population. A *representative sample* is one from which we can draw accurate, unbiased estimates of the characteristics of the larger population. The validity of an audit project depends in part on how the sample is selected. There are two groups of sampling methods known as probability and non-probability sampling.

Probability sampling

When probability sampling is used it is possible to specify the probability of a particular individual in the population being included in the sample. In its simplest form each individual has the same probability of being included in the sample. The three commonly used methods of probability sampling are simple random sampling, systematic sampling and stratified sampling.

Simple random sampling involves randomly selecting a given number from a list of all the population. It may be useful to use a list of random numbers which can be found in most statistics textbooks and on many computer packages. Patients might be identified using a random selection of hospital numbers. Alternatively, a list of all those eligible may be prepared and numbers allocated to them, from which a random selection can be made. You could even choose to draw names out of a hat.

Systematic sampling involves selecting the first individual to be included at random and then the rest of the sample at a fixed interval after the first. For example, the twelfth patient admitted within a certain time-frame was selected randomly then every sixth patient after that. The size of the interval is determined by the size of the population divided by the size of the sample needed.

Stratified random sampling is used to ensure certain groups of the population are represented in the sample. The sample is divided into groups or strata who share the same characteristics, for example gender, age, or postal code. Then a random sample is selected from each strata. If the population is clinical staff your strata might then include doctors (senior house officers, registrars, consultants); nurses (staff nurses, ward managers). In order to be representative the number randomly selected for the sample is in proportion to the numbers in each strata.

Non-probability sampling

With non-probability sampling the team have no way of knowing the probability that an individual will be chosen for the sample, so there is no way of determining how representative the sample is. There are three main methods of non-probability sampling: purposive sampling, convenience sampling and quota sampling.

Purposive sampling is dependent upon the judgement of the team in determining the individuals or group of individuals to be included in a sample. It is often used with qualitative designs where the audit team are trying to obtain information describing a particular aspect of care and individuals are selected who it is hoped may provide a variety of viewpoints on the topic under review.

Convenience sampling involves selecting those individuals for the sample who are most conveniently available. This might be all in-patients on a ward on a particular day, all patients visiting a surgery in a particular week or the first fifty people in the out-patients waiting area willing to be interviewed.

Quota sampling is convenience sampling in which steps are taken to ensure that certain groups are represented in particular proportions, as in the stratified sample. However, using the population of clinical staff, instead of randomly selecting the representative group a quota sample might include those on duty in a particular week or those first encountered by the auditor and invited to participate.

From the descriptions, we can clearly see that where possible a probability sample gives us a more representative and therefore more valid picture of the entire population. If a list of the population exists then simple random sampling is the method of choice as systematic sampling has the potential to be biased. Stratified random sampling should also be used where possible to ensure that the sample represents the characteristics of the population as a whole, e.g. ethnic groups, gender, age.

Probability sampling methods allow statistical tests of significance to be used, enabling the detection of true difference. This increases the rigour of an audit project. When making the case for change to be made on the basis of audit results it increases the credibility of your case.

Often considerations of time, the availability of appropriate support and the reality of clinical workloads outweigh the advantages of probability sampling. Your audit objective may call for qualitative methods of data collection. It would then be entirely appropriate to use non-probability sampling methods, as in-depth information about an experience will be required rather than information which can be generalised to the population. Whatever methods are chosen by the team, they should be clearly stated with the rationale when reporting the project results to others.

Determining sample size

An important issue to address for any audit project is how large should the study be in order to meet its aim? The idea is that the study should be large enough that we can confidently address the audit objective, but is not too large, thus wasting effort and resource collecting data unnecessarily.

Any clinical audit project collects information from a limited number of subjects, the sample. This information is used to make inferences about what is happening for the whole target population of which the sample is a representative subset. As there is variation within the whole population, it is unlikely, for example, that four samples of 100 patients would each give identical results. We would experience some sample variation.

The idea of sample size calculations is that we make sure our study is large enough that we can be confident that the proportion calculated from the sample would be likely to be within a specified tolerance, say ±1%, of the true population. Most commonly we carry out the calculations so that the word 'likely' means that the sample value will fall within the specified range with probability 0.95. It is possible to change this probability; increasing it to say 0.99 will result in a larger sample size requirement but you will have more confidence in the result. Decreasing the probability will result in a smaller sample size requirement but less confidence in the result.

In order to be able to calculate sample size we need to have a good idea of how often the criteria are met. This may seem strange because it is exactly this proportion that we hope our audit will measure. If we really have no idea how often the criteria are met then we should plan our study for the worst possible scenario, which would be that the criteria are met in only 50% (proportion 0.5) of cases. However, this will lead to an unnecessarily large study if, for example, the proportion meeting the criteria are really say 90%.

Tables 4.1 to 4.3 provide sample size evaluations for the most commonly specified confidence levels, namely 0.90, 0.95 and 0.99.

Table 4.1 **Sample size required if we are to be 90% confident that the sample estimate of proportion meeting criteria are to be within a specified tolerance of the true proportion.**

		Range of likely values (plus and minus)					
		0.01	0.02	0.05	0.1	0.15	0.2
	0.5	6765	1691	271	68	30	17
	0.6	6494	1624	260	65	29	16
The true	0.7	5683	1421	227	57	25	14
value of	0.75	5074	1268	203	51	23	13
proportion	0.8	4330	1082	173	43	19	
adequately	0.85	3450	863	138	35		
managed	0.9	2435	609	97			
	0.95	1285	321				
	0.98	530					
	0.99	268					

Table 4.2 Sample size required if we are to be 95% confident that the sample estimate of proportion meeting criteria are to be within a specified tolerance of the true proportion.

		Range of likely values (plus and minus)					
		0.01	0.02	0.05	0.1	0.15	0.2
	0.5	9604	2401	384	96	43	24
	0.6	9220	2305	369	92	41	23
The true	0.7	8067	2017	323	81	36	20
value of	0.75	7203	1801	288	72	32	18
proportion	0.8	6147	1537	246	61	27	
adequately	0.85	4898	1225	196	49		
managed	0.9	3457	864	138			
	0.95	1825	456				
	0.98	753					
	0.99	380					

Table 4.3 Sample size required if we are to be 99% confident that the sample estimate of proportion meeting criteria are to be within a specified tolerance of the true proportion.

		Range of likely values (plus and minus)					
		0.01	0.02	0.05	0.1	0.15	0.2
	0.5	16 589	4147	664	166	74	41
	0.6	15 926	3981	637	159	71	40
The true	0.7	13 935	3484	557	139	62	35
value of	0.75	12 442	3111	498	124	55	31
proportion	0.8	10 617	2654	425	106	47	
adequately	0.85	8461	2115	338	85		
managed	0.9	5972	1493	239			
	0.95	3152	788				
	0.98	1301					
	0.99	657					

Calculation of sampling size is well described in good statistical texts such as Altman[3], but it may be easier to import a local expert. Strange words and calculations often send those unfamiliar with statistics into blind panic, but it is vital to give adequate time and consideration to determining the right sample if changes in practice are to be made on the basis of their results.

For example, the Scottish Intercollegiate Guidelines Network (SIGN) have produced a guideline entitled 'Obesity in Scotland – integrating prevention with weight management'[4]. A primary health care team wishing to develop these guidelines into a local clinical audit project would need to determine the incidence of overweight patients in their practice population of say 10 000 people. Recent data suggest that on average 44% of adult men in Scotland are overweight, with a body mass index (BMI) 25–29.9, and a further 14% are obese, with a BMI of over 30 (total 58%). Women in Scotland have a lower prevalence of being overweight. On average, 32% of women are overweight and 17% are obese (total 49%).

Using Table 4.4 we can determine the sample size required if we are to be 95% confident that the sample estimate of proportion overweight or obese is to be within a specified tolerance of the true proportion. The expected value is 0.49 for women and 0.58 for men, so looking down the 0.05 column gives us sample sizes of 384 and 369 respectively.

Table 4.4 **Determining sample size.**

		Range of likely values (plus and minus)					
		0.01	0.02	0.05	0.1	0.15	0.2
	0.5	9604	2401	384	96	43	24
	0.6	9220	2305	369	92	41	23
The	**0.7**	8067	2017	323	81	36	20
expected	**0.75**	7203	1801	288	72	32	18
value	**0.8**	6147	1537	246	61	27	
	0.85	4898	1225	196	49		
	0.9	3457	864	138			
	0.95	1825	456				
	0.98	753					
	0.99	380					

If the practice felt that sample sizes of almost 400 were not realistic, one option would be to reduce the level of tolerance they accept to say $\pm$ 0.1, i.e. $\pm$ 10% of the true value, which would take their sample size down below 100. Alternatively, they could reduce the confidence level such that the team can only be 90% confident that the sample will produce a proportion within $\pm$ 0.05 ($\pm$ 5%) of the true value, which will halve the number of people required.

If the sample sizes recommended within Table 4.4 are not realistic for your purposes, you may need to consult someone locally with the necessary expertise to help you decide whether reducing the confidence level or the tolerance would be acceptable within the aims of the project.

If, however, you are using a qualitative approach to collecting data you are likely to be looking at non-probability sampling. For example, a project looking at uptake and duration of breastfeeding might wish to complement data collection on breastfeeding rates with some focus groups looking at advice received and the factors influencing women's decisions. A random sample of those choosing to breastfeed, and another of those choosing artificial methods, could be approached and asked to join focus groups. Alternatively, volunteers to participate in focus groups could be found using local new parent newsletters. The sample would then consist of enough women to participate in focus groups to ensure that the range of views had been included; from women choosing to breastfeed, choosing not to breastfeed and women from ethnic minority groups.

Find out what resources are available to you locally, in terms of existing data sources, advice and technical support.

Defining the time-frame for data collection

Having determined the sample size, the time-frame can be defined. Hospital information systems may have information about numbers of patients with particular clinical conditions so that you can estimate how long it might take to collect your data.

It is important to consider seasonal variations when defining time-frames for audit as patient populations can vary considerably. During the winter months bronchiolitis is responsible for many admissions to paediatric medical wards which might need to be taken into consideration for an audit on cross infection in paediatrics. During the summer months many areas of the country find that their population increases vastly with tourists – an audit of admissions to accident and emergency may look very different according to the seasons and this would need to be considered when deciding on a time-frame for data collection.

Who should collect data?

Having determined the sample size and time-frame, the team identify specific individuals to take responsibility for collecting and collating the audit data. This may be just one person or it may be a group of people, who are referred to as the *auditors*. In order for them to retain the ownership of the standard, it is essential that the group decides who should take on the role of auditor.

The auditor is the person whom the group feels would be most appropriate to audit the standard, though they need not be a member of the group. This obviously depends on the nature of the project. For example, if one of the structure criteria states that nursing staff possess an agreed level of knowledge and understanding about a particular subject area, the auditor has to be someone who is capable of assessing the knowledge levels and who is both acceptable and non-threatening to staff.

By contrast, a team looking at patient privacy and dignity may feel that as health professionals they are too comfortable in a hospital setting to be objective about the experience of being a patient. They therefore ask the patient representative on the group to be the auditor.

The choice of auditor may also depend on the group's level of trust and maturity with clinical audit. At first most professional groups wish to be responsible for measuring their own practice. As confidence grows, staff may invite others to provide a more objective view; nursing staff from one ward collecting data for another; even a physiotherapist collecting data on the nursing contribution and nurses collecting data on the medical contribution. The group may prefer to enlist the help of clinical audit staff and ask them to collect data. This will depend on the level of support clinical audit staff are able to offer locally.

Once nominated and having agreed to take on the role, the auditor assumes responsibility for collecting and collating the audit data.

Staff and patient consent

The consent of all those involved in providing data should also be sought before data collection takes place. Consent and confidentiality are discussed in more detail in Chapter 7 in the section on clinical audit and ethical issues. A system for ensuring that staff and patients are given the opportunity to opt out of involvement in audit is essential. A code of conduct for collection of data directly from patients or others via interview or questionnaire can be found in Appendix 1.

It is important to let staff know that data collection will be taking place so that they can ask questions and clarify any difficulties they may have. The usual communication channels can be used to this end – notice boards, meetings, team briefing. If a staff member is anxious about having their practice scrutinised it is important to take time to reassure them that audit is about the development of patient care and not the inspection or criticism of individual staff. As previously discussed, within a culture of trust and support, clinical audit has the potential to empower and develop staff.

What information is given to patients about audit in your workplace? What could be done to improve it?

Recording audit data

Data collection sheets are normally devised as the measurement tool is developed. If you have access to specialist audit software packages these may be generated for you. As previously mentioned, the methods for analysis of data should be planned from the outset and this may influence the way in which data are recorded. Audit records can also be generated using word processing packages and spreadsheet packages such as Microsoft Excel. Piloting your audit tool gives you the opportunity to check that your data collection sheets or audit records are set out appropriately with adequate space in each section for auditors to record the necessary information.

Data needs to be collected such that no individual patient or staff member can be identified. It needs to be anonymised. It may be helpful to devise a coding system known only to the auditors.

You may wish to set an expected compliance rate or target. You may have considered this already whilst determining your sample size. Comparing the actual with the expected level of compliance allows the auditor to see at a glance areas where achievement is good, or areas where the results are lower than expected.

The following example illustrates a process of careful planning and preparation before data collection takes place.

Acute pain management project

Michele Hiscock, Nurse Consultant, Practice Development & Quality, Royal Brompton Hospital

This project to improve surgical acute pain management has been running since 1992 and has resulted in the development of an Acute Pain service.

The professional groups involved in acute pain management were invited to develop a standard and audit tool. These professionals include physiotherapists, nurses, pharmacists and doctors in the hospital. Once the standard was approved by the team and others within the organisation the audit was conducted by the multidisciplinary staff amongst their daily duties. This has continued on a yearly basis. The data are collected over a month, which is negotiated with the clinical areas so that only one audit is being conducted at the one time. This is also to ensure that the Systems Administrator for the Dynamic Quality Improvement (DQI) Programme is able to maintain an efficient system of audit analysis. Staff audit their own practices; for example, the physiotherapists ask the patient 'Are you able to perform shoulder and arm exercises with pain at an acceptable level?' To improve inter-rater reliability a meeting is held before the audit to read through each question and agree on what should be a Yes/No/Not applicable answer. The auditors are the representatives from the area/profession who attend the pain meetings.

The number of patients audited is based on a 10% convenience sample of the number of surgical operations performed over a one month period. This information is obtained from the Master Scheduler in theatres. Staff and patients are invited to take part in the audit; there is no record of anyone refusing to take part.

There have not been any problems collecting the data that are related to the methodology itself. However, auditors have found the audit time-consuming on occasions when the wording of some criteria are not in lay terms. An example of this is 'Did you feel that the nurse understood your perception of pain?' The auditor has to explain to some patients what perception of pain means.

When using not applicable (N/A) we have found that an explanation for this is very useful. For example, when assessing and documenting the patient's history of pain when nothing was documented the auditors wrote N/A. If it was blank it should have been No, as there was no evidence to suggest the patient was asked whether they did or did not have a history of pain.

Qualitative information has proved valuable in understanding the reasons for a low or high compliance. An example of this is when a patient was asked 'Were you involved with your pain assessment?'. The patient said 'Yes, but I lied about my pain scores'. He then explained that his mother had recently died of cancer and she had received morphine for pain relief. The patient was recovering from a thoracotomy and received morphine for pain relief. When he discovered this he lied about his scores as he believed that it was the morphine that killed his mother, not cancer.

We have explored audit results by carrying out point prevalence studies. An example of this is when we asked in the audit criteria 'Did you feel that your mobility was restricted by pain in the:

a. chest
b. leg
c. elsewhere.

The compliance for c. was 74% ($n = 44/59$); from the qualitative comments we found that 6 of these patients had pain in their neck. We wanted to explore why these patients had neck pain so devised a point prevalence tool with multidisciplinary input. We asked 12 questions which included if they had neck pain was it left, right, back or front. Did they have necklines in situ? If yes, how many and what side? Did they have a previous history of pain in their neck? Our results showed that all of the patients that had neck pain had a previous history of either whiplash injuries, arthritis or spondylitis, none of which had been documented in the medical notes.

This information would have been important for the anaesthetist when inducing the patient and for the recovery and intensive care staff nursing the unconscious patient. As a result of this, when the standard was redefined, we added 'neck' and 'elsewhere' to the audit question.

Until 1997 we had protocols for pain management in each of the clinical areas; now we have one standard which encompasses all areas. This cuts down on the length of time spent auditing. It also makes action planning more beneficial by improving the service throughout the hospital.

Comparison and analysis

Having collected the audit data, the next stage involves collating it and analysing the responses in preparation for feedback. The method of analysis will depend on the type of data you have generated, as illustrated in Table 4.5 (adapted from Donnan[5]).

Table 4.5 **Types of data**

Type	Description	Examples
Categorical	Nominal: data in separate classes which have no numerical relationship	Gender, yes/no answers, ward
	Ordinal: data in separate classes with order relationship	Degrees of pain, social class, level of agreement with a statement
Numerical	Discrete: arise from counts or scales	Number of non-attenders at a clinic, score on a visual analogue scale
	Continuous measurements: can take any value in range	Height, weight, haemoglobin level

The first step in data analysis is to collate and describe it. The commonest ways of describing and displaying data are in the form of tables and charts, examples of which are on the following pages. You may choose to display results against expected outcome, current data against previous data sets, or data from one clinical unit against data from another. You will need to be aware of other (confounding) variables influencing these comparisons such as staffing levels, case mix.

Pie chart

This is suitable for displaying nominal or ordinal data. It involves dividing a circle into wedges according to the proportion of the category the wedge represents. The more of the category present the bigger the slice of pie.

Figure 4.1 shows a pie chart for the percentage of different diagnostic tests required at an out-patient clinic. This was a part of a clinical audit project which improved the time patients had to wait for results of commonly requested diagnostic tests (Morris-Thompson[6]).

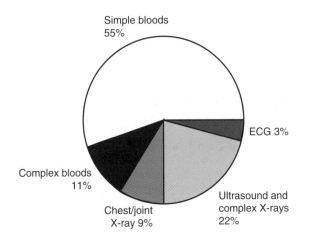

Figure 4.1 **Pie chart showing out-patient test requirement (Morris-Thompson[5]).**

Bar chart

This is another suitable means of displaying nominal or ordinal data. For each category a bar is drawn which equals the frequency or percentage of that category. Conventionally there are gaps between the bars to indicate that these are discrete categories. Bars may be drawn horizontally or vertically and the frequency axis should start from zero. Figure 4.2 shows the results of a project to implement national guidelines for the management of pain in children (Buchanan et al[7]). Data have been collected on three occasions and the bar chart clearly illustrates the improvement in evaluation, i.e. reassessment of pain levels 30 minutes after intervention and documentation of the child's response to the intervention.

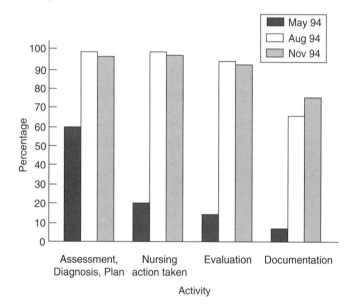

Figure 4.2 **Activities being performed at different time points (Buchanan et al[7]).**

Histogram

This is suitable for displaying numerical data and cannot be used for nominal or ordinal data. The range for the variable is divided into intervals of equal width and the number in each interval calculated. Bars are then drawn of height equal to the frequency or percentage for the interval. There are no gaps between the bars because the measurements are on a numerical scale. Figure 4.3 shows a histogram of the ages of patients diagnosed with epilepsy as a part of a primary/secondary care interface audit on the management of patients with epilepsy in Cumbria (Hargreaves[8]).

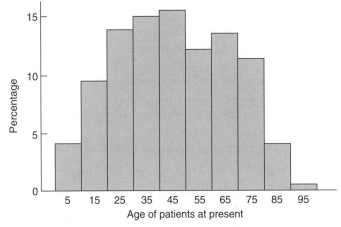

Figure 4.3 **Histogram of age of patients with epilepsy (Hargreaves[8]).**

Histograms are often used to judge whether data are normally distributed. The normal distribution is symmetrical and has a characteristic bell shape.

It may well be appropriate to do some more in-depth analysis to make inferences from your data by applying appropriate statistical tests. This is where good planning is essential. If statistical tests are to be applied, the measurement tools and sample size need to be designed accordingly. You may wish to see whether changes in practice occurring as a result of the project have produced improvements which are statistically significant. Again, this is an area where you may be able to draw on the skills within the team or a local statistician. You might have access to computer software packages such as SPSS, or Epi Info. These packages can provide invaluable help at this stage.

A note of caution – computer software packages are good at calculating statistics and can produce wonderfully impressive numbers. However, in the hands of the inexperienced there is a serious risk of producing wonderfully impressive nonsense!

Your data may also consist of qualitative, descriptive elements; for example, comments, transcribed interviews, notes from focus groups. There are a number of ways of approaching it. The data need to be simplified in some way. This may involve some form of coding or a process of extracting particular excerpts which describe issues of importance to the data provider. You need to first read and reread the data. You then need to simplify it, either by imposing a framework on the data, or allowing the themes to emerge from the words of the data providers whilst suspending your own views.

Miles and Huberman[9] describe a three stage process of data reduction, data display and conclusions and verification. Data reduction involves summarising, coding and dividing into themes, clusters or categories. Again this is a skilled activity and may require the input of an expert.

Practical suggestions for qualitative data analysis:

- Use post-it notes to cluster comments together.
- Different coloured highlighter pens can be useful to pick out data on different themes.
- Cut up narrative data and rearrange into themes using scissors and glue or cut and paste on a computer.

An example is shown in Box 4.1 using extracts looking at barriers to clinical audit[10]. Interviewees had been asked to identify what they perceived to be barriers to the further development of clinical audit in their workplace. The raw data consisted of 28 interview transcripts all of which mentioned lack of time.

Box 4.1 Coding responses

How did respondents describe their lack of time?	Code
We have had improvements, but we could have a lot more if we had more time …	More improvements if time
Clinical audit is a very time-consuming process, we can't afford that number of people, that amount of time …	Takes people away from work
We have no time, our typical daily workload is ten in, ten out and ten for theatres.	Workload
Clinical audit is yet another thing to find time for.	Yet another thing

Box 4.1 Coding responses (contd.)

How did respondents describe their lack of time?	Code
On the wards the staff are under so much pressure they lose sight of the passion for what they are doing.	Pressure of work
Staff were so stressed and busy clinical audit wasn't the highest thing on their agenda.	Staff are stressed

The codes on the right in Box 4.1 can then be clustered, drawing together words that are conveying a similar idea. These can then be brought into the audit summary and discussed with the team.

An audit summary form can be found in Appendix 3 and may be helpful when communicating results to the rest of the team. This takes us into the fourth phase of the clinical audit cycle, that of *planning and implementing action to improve quality*.

Find a clinical audit project report in a journal and display the results using a chart or graph.

Summary

- The third phase of the quality improvement cycle is the measuring phase, which involves comparing existing practice against your criteria.
- Methods of data collection are carefully considered and existing data used where possible.
- Measurement involves calculating a representative sample which may need expert advice.
- The group needs to decide who will collect data. This person should be capable, acceptable and non-threatening to patients and staff.
- The consent of patients and staff should be considered before data collection begins.
- Results can be simply displayed using a range of charts and diagrams.

References

1. Russell IT, Wilson BJ 1992 Audit the third clinical science? Quality in Health Care 1(1): 51–55
2. Cook P 1996 Audit methodology: time for a rethink? Network issue no. 22, pp 6–8
3. Altman DG 1991 Practical statistics for medical research. Chapman and Hall, London
4. SIGN 1996 Obesity in Scotland: Integrative prevention with weight management. A national clinical guideline recommended for use in Scotland by the Scottish Intercollegiate Guidelines Network (SIGN Publication No. 8). SIGN, Edinburgh
5. Donnan P 1996 Quantitative analysis. In: Cormack D (ed) The research process in Nursing. Blackwell, Oxford
6. Morris Thompson T 1996 Implementing a near patient test facility. Journal of the Association of Quality in Healthcare 3(3): 110–117
7. Buchanan L, Voigtman J, Mills H 1997 Implementing the AHCPR Pain Management Pediatric Guideline in a multicultural practice setting. Journal of Nursing Care Quality 1(3): 23–35
8. Hargreaves C 1994 The management of patients with epilepsy. Network issue no. 15, pp 10–12
9. Miles MB, Huberman AM 1994 Qualitative data analysis: an expanded sourcebook. Sage, London
10. Morrell C, Harvey G, Kitson AL 1995 The reality of practitioner based quality improvement, report no. 14. National Institute for Nursing, Oxford

5
Planning for improvement

This chapter covers:

- feedback and evaluation
- agreeing the appropriate course of action
- managing change
- re-audit and evaluation
- regular re-audit and review
- lessons learned
- report writing
- presentation skills
- review and assessment of existing clinical audit projects.

Feedback and evaluation

Once an audit summary is complete, the auditor then feeds back the findings to the clinical audit group for interpretation. The auditor should not make interpretations without consulting and involving the group. It is essential that the audit summary should provide constructive feedback by reporting on areas of both high and low achievement. The group can then discuss why some areas have been more successful and how to extend any high achievement to the other areas considered.

Sharing the results of clinical audit can be perceived as threatening to staff. Information needs to be communicated in a way that respects confidentiality and is sensitive to individual needs. The clinical audit group take responsibility for communicating the results to the professional groups they represent and asking for the comments of those involved to help with interpretation and action planning.

Where results show areas of excellent practice it is good to take the time to congratulate those involved and to celebrate success. Too often the emphasis in clinical audit is placed on the areas where further work is required and the good practice is ignored. The clinical audit group can then discuss and interpret the findings further and begin to clarify the areas where action is required to improve the level of achievement.

A systematic process needs to be applied to the planning and implementation of the necessary changes in practice identified.

Agreeing the appropriate course of action

This is the phase of clinical audit where many teams run into difficulties. Results clearly show that problems exist, but acting upon that information to improve care is a complex undertaking. For this reason the next section outlines some theories of change to help unravel the issues which need to be considered when embarking on a process of action planning. An example action plan form is shown in Appendix 3; this acts as a focus for the team, to document what they have planned.

The action plan needs careful consideration and for each issue identified will include:

- *The appropriate course of action* – having identified the priorities for action these need to be clearly documented.
- *A named person responsible for the action* – it is important that the group identifies a named individual/s to be responsible for leading or coordinating each of the actions specified. Most of the clinical audit group will have responsibility for some aspect of the plan depending on their particular skills and the professional group that they represent.
- *The time-scale for action* – the group need to determine how long they need to implement each of the actions identified. This depends on the nature of the problem and the type of action required. *Short-term actions* are those which can be remedied almost immediately, in less than 6 weeks. *Medium term actions* require a longer period of up to 6 months to implement, while *long-term actions* are those that will take over 6 months to achieve.

Example

An audit conducted in a nursing home of the Nutritional Standards of Care for the Older Adult revealed that a number of actions needed to be taken. These included:

- *short-term actions* such as weighing patients once a month
- *medium-term actions* such as undertaking a nutritional risk assessment on all patients and
- *long-term actions*, which involved building a new kitchen.

Before the action plan is drawn up it is worth considering the wider issues involved so that the plan reflects the careful consideration of potential barriers to improving care.

Managing change

In order to effectively plan and implement changes in practice it can be useful to consider the process in the context of a model or framework. These ideas may be useful as you plan the implementation of best practice as well as at the stage of planning improvement. There are five important factors to consider (Fig. 5.1)[1]:

- change strategies and theories
- the change itself
- the environment or setting in which change will occur
- those involved in changing their practice
- the use of change agents.

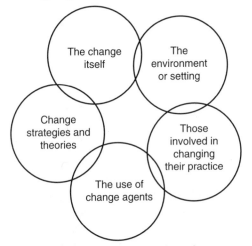

Figure 5.1 **Points to consider in managing change.**

Change strategies and theories

It can be helpful to identify the strategy you intend to use to implement change. Using a theoretical framework to reflect upon your situation may clarify the way in which you decide to proceed. There are numerous theories in relation to the nature of change and why change does or does not occur.

Systems theory offers an interpretation of why and how change occurs. One of the most well known theories is based on the notion that people, teams and organisations are interdependent or interconnected and that behaviour is derived from the connections. Within this 'force field' of relationships three main phases are outlined which need to occur for change to take place[2].

1. **Unfreeze** – where the individual or organisation begins to move from the status quo. At this stage the present conditions may be critically analysed.
2. **Move** – in this phase three potential situations can arise:
   a. equilibrium where there is no change
   b. the driving forces (positive factors) being greater than the restraining forces (moving towards your goal)
   c. the restraining forces (negative factors) being greater than the driving forces (moving away from your goal).
3. **Re-freeze** – this stage is about stabilising the change and using new knowledge.

Unfreezing usually happens during the defining and measuring phase of the clinical audit cycle. Practitioners have their awareness of the issues under review raised, and the status quo is questioned as baseline data are collected. Once action is planned and implemented it is important to plan for re-freezing by allocating the time and resources to see the changes made established into routine practice.

Another useful model identifies three strategies for effecting change[3]:

- *Empirical-rational strategies* assume that people are rational and logical in their actions, therefore if research suggests a particular practice is best, staff will adopt it.
- *Normative-re-educative strategies* assume that people's attitudes, values, beliefs and relationships affect their behaviour and the way they act upon information and knowledge.
- *Power-coercive approaches* depend on the use of power or authority in some form. Change occurs when those with less power act on the directives of those in a leadership position, for example as a result of health policy decisions.

It is most appropriate to use a normative-re-educative approach to change within an improvement-based approach to clinical audit (see Chapter 1). This approach views staff as partners in the change process and values their contribution.

There are other models of change you may wish to consider. One alternative[4] comprises three phases: analysis of the *environment*, i.e. culture, stakeholder expectations, resources and capability; *choice* – in terms of identifying options, evaluating them and selecting a strategy; and *implementation* – planning, structuring and managing the change.

These models can also be helpful when considering the other four factors described in the interlocking circles, by linking the factors together into a coherent plan.

The change itself

The change itself is likely to be dynamic and multifaceted. The course of action that needs to be taken may not be immediately obvious. By the same token the immediately obvious course of action may not be the most effective. There may be several possible routes to achieve the desired change and the task of the group is to identify the alternatives and prioritise action. The group members interpret the problems identified in the audit and consider each one individually, discussing possible ways of addressing the problem. There are a number of group techniques for problem-solving, decision-making and consensus development which you might find useful in this prioritising process. Some of them are outlined below.

'*Quick think*' is used to free up people's ideas and to help them to think in new ways. The facilitator encourages people to explore an issue by sharing their first response. Each suggestion is recorded, however odd, wild or impossible it may seem (good ideas sometimes have these characteristics when first conceived). The facilitator does not allow any 'for and against' discussion or value judgments to take place. When no more ideas are forthcoming, the facilitator helps the group to look at all the contributions and engage in discussion. Eventually, ideas considered to be worth further exploration are prioritised. 'Quick think' is usually very lively and fun.

Force field analysis is a technique to help people to look at the driving and restraining forces acting on a situation. Driving forces are factors which indicate instability and an openness to change; they are positive forces for change. Restraining forces are those which promote stability and maintain the status quo, indicating resistance to change. The facilitator writes 'Driving forces' at one side of a flipchart sheet, 'Current situation' in the middle and 'Restraining forces' at the other side (Fig. 5.2). Group members are invited to make suggestions as to what the driving and restraining forces might be which are put up on the flipchart.

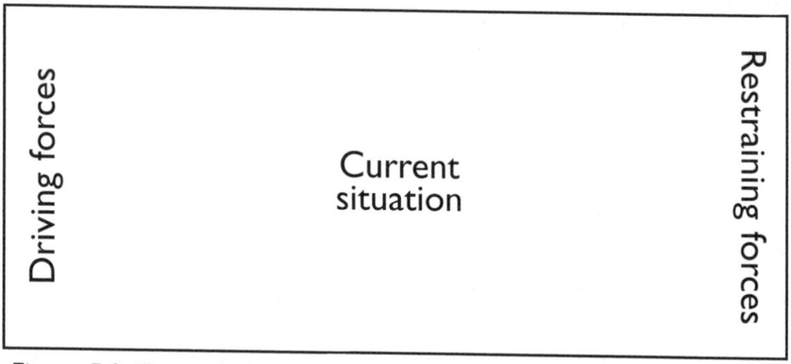

Figure 5.2 **Force field analysis.**

The forces are then analysed by the group to determine the needs and priorities to be addressed in planning for change.

SWOT analysis is a similar technique to the force field analysis in that it is also a method for identifying factors which promote and oppose change. In this case, four key dimensions are studied: Strengths, Weaknesses, Opportunities and Threats – hence the reference to 'SWOT' analysis. Strengths and weaknesses are internal, i.e. characteristics of the initiative under review, and opportunities and threats are external, i.e. environmental factors which will affect the development of the initiative. The facilitator divides the board or flipchart paper into four squares and heads each square with one of the key headings, as illustrated in Figure 5.3.

STRENGTHS	WEAKNESSES
OPPORTUNITIES	THREATS

Figure 5.3 **SWOT analysis.**

Group members then suggest ideas under each of the headings, either in a large group, or by breaking into smaller subgroups, depending on the numbers involved.

Nominal group technique helps a group to move towards a
consensus, either in terms of making a position statement or
making a decision. It can be used, for example, to reach agreement after a 'quick think' exercise, to establish the needs and
priorities for change identified previously in a force field analysis or to reach agreement on a shared philosophy. The facilitator invites each member of the group to put forward his or her
views on the topic under discussion. 'Going round the group' is
an effective way of making sure that everyone contributes. Each
person's statement is written on the flipchart and discussion is
kept to a minimum at that point. When all views have been
recorded, each statement is discussed in turn. Only those statements with which *everyone* agrees are retained, the others are
scrapped.

This technique can be combined with multi-voting so that
after the discussion each participant has a set number of votes
to allocate to the ideas put forward. They may choose to allocate all their votes to one idea or divide them between those
considered priorities. This leaves the group with a list of ideas
ranked in order of priority.

Snowballing is another way of reaching consensus and ensuring that even the most reticent group members contribute. The
facilitator asks the group to divide into pairs and to discuss the
topic for a timed period. The length of time for discussion will
vary according to group size and how much time is available.
The pair are asked to identify areas where they can reach agreement. The facilitator is the time-keeper and tells the pair to join
with another, when the time is up. In fours, each pair shares
with the other the consensus statements. All the statements are
discussed for a timed period and those with which all four agree
are retained. The process is repeated with the four joining up
with another four, then eight with eight and so on, until the
group has become one again. By this time, consensus statements
will have been agreed by the whole group.

These techniques enable the group to consider actions which
need to be taken in the context of the wider organisation. The
third factor needing to be addressed is the environment or setting affected by the planned action. There may be wider issues

which have not already been highlighted and so reflecting on the environment is essential to the careful planning of change.

The environment or setting in which the change will occur

There are a number of issues affecting the way in which a change can be introduced including:

- Culture – this is a wide ranging concept and needs to take into account the values of society, the influence of health policy, the values of the organisation often manifest in the management style, and sensitivity to the values and ethnicity of the target population.
- Systems and structures – when planning change it is important to identify who the stakeholders are and how they can be influenced. What is the management structure and how is it most effectively utilised to support change? What systems of communication exist within the organisation to effect change (newsletters, meetings, bulletins, team briefing)? Are there procedures within the organisation which need to be gone through when introducing something new?
- Learning environment – in some organisations professional development and learning in teams is encouraged and seen as an everyday part of practice. Within such an environment proposed improvements are taken on board more easily than in a setting where learning and development are not regarded as important.
- Resources – it is useful to identify resources available to support change when planning action. Resources to consider include staff who may act as change agents, administrative support, existing communication channels. You may also be in need of physical or financial resources and your audit results may help in the negotiation to secure these.

It can be helpful when considering the setting of a planned change to think in terms of systems, to look at how structures, resources and culture are connected. It may be useful to map the connections rather than focus on individual aspects. 'Systems thinking is a discipline for seeing wholes. It is a framework for seeing patterns of change rather than static snapshots.'[5] Systemic thinking is also a very useful way of considering those who are affected by the proposed change – looking at their relationships rather than at staff members in isolation.

Those involved in changing their practice

People have all sorts of reasons to change or not to change their behaviour. Each staff member affected by proposed changes in practice will have their own particular set of values, attitudes and beliefs which will influence whether or not they are willing to take on board something new. Within a clinical team you will find a range of reactions to proposed change and it has been suggested that people fall into the following groups[6]:

Innovators	proactive during the process of change
Early adopters	readily accept change
Early majority	first group to follow the early adopter
Later majority	other groups follow suit
Laggards	reticent group who remain sceptical
Rejecters	openly oppose the change

By identifying the fact that they are likely to encounter resistance at the planning stage the clinical audit group can prepare themselves to support colleagues through the transition. Commonly, people resist change because they perceive that it will increase their workload or change their working relationships. It is important to hear these issues and work to support staff through the transition. This is the role of the change agent – to act as a catalyst in the team, enabling change to happen.

The use of change agents

Staff rarely change their behaviour on the basis of a memo or written instruction. It is most often as a result of a conversation where a respected colleague has listened to their doubts and persuaded them of the merits of change. These respected colleagues are often known as opinion leaders[7]. You may, however, need the assistance of a variety of change agents when implementing an action plan from a clinical audit project.

- Good managers – who empower, enable and encourage staff to adopt new practice by their support.
- Opinion leaders – who implement change with enthusiasm, leading by example and taking time to persuade the cynics in the team. A review of the literature suggests that opinion leaders have the following characteristics: influential, respected individuals, clinical experts, high social status, centre of interpersonal networks, articulate, accessible and

approachable, willing to share knowledge, like to teach, have current and up to date knowledge[8].

- Facilitators – a clinical audit group facilitator will adopt a number of roles during the course of a project (see Chapter 8) and it will normally include that of change agent. Using his or her skills with groups and individuals the facilitator may be the ideal person to ensure that everyone's doubts are heard and to provide extra support through the process of change.
- Innovators – clinical staff who readily embrace new initiatives and carry their peer group with them, they may not be as influential as the opinion leaders but contribute to the critical mass necessary for change to be established in the practice of a team.

For a change in practice you have identified in your unit, draw up an action plan to prioritise your actions, and consider what change management models will help to guide the planning process.

Action planning or 'Eating an elephant one bite at a time'

Lorraine Hughes, Practice Development Nurse; Jill Regan, Ward Sister, Orthopaedics (nursing documentation group leader); Kevin Randall, Staff Nurse, Accident and Emergency (part-time project leader), Bridgend & District NHS Trust

During the early part of the 1980s the 'Nursing Process' was introduced within Wales. In support of this initiative an 'All Wales' recording format was produced which included separate sections for demographic details, initial assessment, the care planned and a summary sheet. With the exception of the section for demographic details, all other sections are either blank or contain broad prompts.

The problems – the nursing record

The documentation that was being used in the Surgical Directorate had not been reviewed since its introduction in 1982. The majority of nurses were vaguely discontented about the length of time taken to record care and some were uncertain as to whether they recorded the right sort of information, even after years of experience. This feeling had increased with the rising number of complaints and difficulties encountered in ascertaining what actually had happened during the course of a patient's stay. However, no one really seemed to know where to start or what to do to improve the situation.

Problem clarification

During 1996, a Trust-wide project was commenced to attempt to develop Corporate Nursing Standards and the topics included:

- nutrition
- continence promotion
- pressure sore prevention
- moving and handling
- wound care
- pain management
- nursing documentation.

Nursing records were used as the basis for auditing whether clinically effective care was being delivered. The criteria used were:

1. Evidence of comprehensive initial assessment.
2. Identified problems on admission are acted upon.
3. Risk factors are identified.

The findings of the initial audit concluded that:

- The documentation format was not conducive to the effective recording of assessments and intervention, encouraging fragmentation and duplication.
- If the record did not contain a preprinted model then limited assessment occurred. Only 38% of a sample of 121 patient records received a comprehensive assessment.
- Problems identified on initial assessment were not included in care plans.
- Problems documented as resolved in the office record remained problems on the care plan.

What do we do to improve the situation?

Create a communication structure:

1. Reports and presentations of findings to ward sisters.
2. Reports to Executive Nurse and Management Executive.
3. Consolidate previously existing link groups for corporate standards by asking ward sisters to lead a group.

4. Create a post for part-time release from clinical practice for a project manager.
5. Agree an action plan.
6. Try to get some funding.

Now that we had clearly identified the problems the next task was to decide what type of nursing record should replace the old one. Should we design one locally or try to find one that had already been tried and tested? The senior nurse for surgery had visited a neighbouring Trust where a 3 year project had been undertaken to develop a multi-professional record for use in any health care setting. The sister leading the Nursing Documentation Link Group and the Practice Development Nurse for the Trust visited the Project Leader of the neighbouring Trust, who generously offered support and guidance to our plans for implementation. A staff nurse from our Accident and Emergency Department was released for one day per week to oversee the project.

A lengthy process of consultation about the new document was undertaken, initially planned to be 3 months, but eventually taking 8 months. Just when you think everyone is clear about everything, you accidentally discover they aren't! Each area was represented in the link group and link nurses were asked to discuss the draft document with their own ward-based team, propose amendments and feed back in link group meetings. Attendance was sometimes a problem. To try to improve the problem two actions were taken:

- A summary of the role and responsibilities of a link nurse.
- Attendance was monitored by the group and project leader and if two consecutive meetings were missed the senior nurse for surgery sent the individual a letter reminding them of their responsibilities.

The initial audit had been undertaken in April 1997. The new draft document was introduced for discussion in August 1997 and re-audit still using the original record was undertaken in October 1997, the results of which were very encouraging. So much so, that some discussions occurred regarding whether a new record was necessary. Best laid plans ... good communication works wonders in itself!

The consultation period came to an end in January 1998 when the document was re-drafted to include assessments which had been developed in various acute settings. The audit revealed that nursing assessment was very different in short stay areas and a suitable record needed to be developed. This proved difficult to agree, due to the tension in finding a balance regarding the extent of assessment and the risks of undertaking a less than comprehensive assessment. The lack of an appropriate model for short stay patients was the key issue. Agreement was eventually reached based on a document which was devised in our day care unit with extended sections to cover care up to 48 hours.

The pilot

Only two wards piloted the record with multi-professional involvement. The remaining two wards, one orthopaedic and one general surgery, implemented the record for use by the nursing team, but with a view to multi-professional involvement at a later date. The pilot study commenced in February 1998. The corporate standards audit took place less than one month after implementation and the nurses were concerned that due to the major change in the document the results would be adversely affected. Not so – the results continued to show an improvement in all aspects of care – contrary to the published evidence regarding change management, i.e. don't audit too soon after a major change.

It was during this period that the most meaningful amendments occurred to the document. Meetings were held each week by the project leader specifically for nurses to discuss problems they had as individuals in using the format and most of the teaching and problem-solving were covered in these sessions.

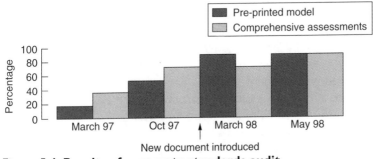

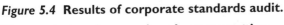

Figure 5.4 **Results of corporate standards audit.**

The next step for nursing documentation

- The document will need an annual review as it must always be able to reflect the changing needs of our patients and services.
- Staged progression according to the capabilities of individual wards will be respected.

- We still need to consider how to improve care planning aspects of the document. Although duplication between the 'office record' and the care plan has been dramatically reduced, the framework for planning care still lacks structure and remains confusing as to what should be written where.

The next step for multi-professional documentation

In areas where multi-professional involvement in the record is apparent, all the professions involved feel that communication is much improved:

—The record is shared amongst physiotherapists, occupational therapists, dietitians and nurses.
—Time spent explaining patient problems to one another is much less.
—All the information for each patient is kept in one record.
—Medical staff read the record more often as it is current and comprehensive.

Lessons learned about action planning

- Don't underestimate the courage it takes to publicise adverse findings.
- Changing practice takes longer than you think.
- Make sure the problem is clearly identified; use a few meaningful criteria to audit – too many generate confusing data. People will see the need to change and participate more willingly.
- Ensure that reports go to all the right people. It increases everyone's accountability to actively *do* something toward the planned improvement.
- Create a solid communication structure and make sure everyone is clear about their roles and responsibilities.
- Be prepared to change your plans as you understand the problem more clearly and more people become involved.
- Re-audit regularly – the best part is being able to demonstrate the actual improvement – to everyone.
- Use the whole process to help staff to develop problem-solving and change management skills – create opportunities.
- Don't reinvent the wheel.
- Be prepared to take risks – don't get scared – the bigger the problem the easier it is to demonstrate improvement.
- Make positive change a priority.

Re-audit and evaluation

Taking into account the actions to be implemented and the time-scale for these, the group sets a date to re-audit the standard. This should be after the deadline for the most long-term action to be implemented. Comparing the first and second set of audit results will then enable the group to evaluate what improvements have been made and possible areas where further action is required.

On completing the re-auditing stage, the group will have moved through the complete clinical audit cycle. Depending on the results obtained, they must then agree on their next course of action, which may involve one of several possible steps:

- If problems remain or new problems are identified, the group plan further action and re-audit as before.
- If they are achieving the standard, the group may elect to raise the expected level of achievement of the standard in order to aim for further improvement.
- If the standard reflects best practice, the group may set a timetable for regular re-audit and review of the standard.

Regular re-audit and review

How often to re-audit and review clinical audit projects is a matter for local decision. Re-audit needs to become part of routine practice integral to the organisation's clinical audit strategy and annual planning process. It is usual to re-audit every 6 months or annually. Time-frames should be decided by the group and according to the topic but the following issues should be considered:

- the workload of auditors
- the number of other projects being regularly re-audited
- other regular monitoring activities
- maintaining staff interest and awareness.

The objective and criteria need to be regularly reviewed to keep in step with the evidence. If standards are taken from national guidelines, which are usually updated every 2 years, they should be reviewed accordingly. Where standards are based on systematic reviews of research evidence these reviews are also regularly updated by their authors and again standards should be reviewed to reflect any new information.

Where other research evidence or expert consensus is used as the evidence base this should be reviewed annually by searching and appraising the most recent literature, to ensure that your standard remains as current as possible.

Lessons learned

It is important to consider the less measurable results of a clinical audit project. Once the clinical audit group have completed the cycle it is worth taking some time to reflect upon the process and identify the lessons learned. The following questions could provide a starting point for discussion:

- What have been the benefits of involvement in the project?
- What problems have been encountered and how were they solved?
- What would we do differently next time?
- Are there any issues raised by the project which need further work?
- Were the results worth the cost of the project?
- Has the hard work of the clinical audit group been appreciated by the wider team?

As well as discussing these issues it is useful to document a summary of the discussions to build into your audit report. There are occasions when the audit data do not show significant improvements in patient care but there are intangible benefits of the project for staff, for example increased awareness of a particular issue or improved communication and teamwork. Highlighting these issues is an important part of communicating the benefits of clinical audit to the wider organisation.

Thinking about a clinical audit project you have been involved in, answer the questions above considering the broad benefits of the project to patients, the clinical team and the wider organisation.

Report writing

Increasingly those responsible for funding clinical audit expect detailed written accounts of clinical audit activity. Your organisation may have a standardised proforma for reporting on audit projects; if not, you may find the form in Appendix 3 useful. A full audit project report should include the headings shown in Table 5.1.

Table 5.1 **Headings for an audit report**

Heading	Description
Rationale	Your reasons for choosing the topic
Evidence base	The evidence on which your standard is based
Objective	The objective against which you have compared practice
Involvement	Professional and patient groups involved and consulted
Implementation	The steps you took to implement the standard
Methods	Brief description of audit tool, sample and data collection strategy
Results	Summary of data analysis and changes in practice
Cost	An estimate of the direct costs involved in the project
Lessons learned	Summary of the overall impact of the clinical audit project

You may be asked to write more than one report for a different readership, one for the commissioners, and one for an in-house newsletter. It is therefore important to tailor the information you include to the audience, i.e. to patients and carers, to a professional conference or to the Executive Board. The level of detail and length of the report will also be dictated by who the report is for, but, however brief, you need to communicate enough information so that a reader is left in no doubt as to what you were setting out to do, how you did it and what the results were. You might choose to submit a project report to a journal for publication or a national database in which case you would need to place a particular emphasis on your methods so that others could repeat the project.

Presentation skills

Clinical audit groups are often asked to present their projects to clinical audit steering groups, in-house study days, executive boards or externally at conferences. This can be a daunting prospect, but presentation of your work is an integral part of the project. Good *planning* is essential to good presentation. Just as with report writing, the exact nature of the presentation will depend on the audience. Box 5.1 lists a few practical suggestions for the novice presenter.

Box 5.1 Improving presentation skills

Aims	Be clear about what it is you want to get across and ensure important points are emphasised; be realistic given your allocated time.
Be heard	Make sure that the entire audience can hear you, speak slowly and clearly.
Communicate	This is a two-way process; make eye contact with your audience and draw them in; be aware of your body language.
Delivery	Write a script or set out clear notes and practise to ensure that you stick to time.
Equipment	When using projectors and microphones check that they are in working order and that you are sure how to use the particular model available.
Focus	Audio-visual materials can enhance your presentation by helping the audience to focus on the important points of what you are saying; do not, however, use your slides as your notes, turning away from the audience and saying what they can read for themselves

If members of the clinical audit group choose to do a joint presentation ensure that they rehearse together, as delivery can be ruined by messy changeovers and a lack of clarity over which presenter is saying what. Making presentations is a good way of developing an individual staff member's confidence – for this reason it may be appropriate to encourage an inexperienced member of the team to make a presentation.

Reviewing and assessing an existing clinical audit project

The NHS Executive funded the development of a Clinical Audit Assessment Framework by the Health Services Management Centre (HSMC) at the University of Birmingham[9]. It provides an approach to assessing and improving the effectiveness of clinical audit activities in the NHS, designed for both individual clinical audit projects and entire clinical audit programmes.

The framework for assessing and improving a clinical audit project guides the user to ask three fundamental questions of the project (see Appendix 5 for more detail):

- What are the reasons for doing it?
- What impact does it have?
- What does it cost?

It is suggested that data are collected around these three questions. If the data suggest that the project has not been very effective then the reasons why need to be understood. The project assessment framework identifies six areas for further investigation (Box 5.2).

Box 5.2 Six areas for further investigation

Efforts to understand problems and improve future performance should focus on:
- objectives
- involvement
- use of evidence
- project management
- methods
- evaluation.

Careful interpretation of this information is needed to form the basis for an action plan to prevent similar problems occurring in future. An assessment framework form has been developed to help the process and can be found in Appendix 5.

Try filling in the form in Appendix 5 for a project that has been completed in your area recently. Reflect upon any difficulties you encounter.

Summary

- The fourth phase, *taking action to improve*, is vital for effecting change.
- Once the audit data have been analysed, the group agree appropriate courses of action for the problems identified.
- The group then identify named individuals to be responsible for leading or coordinating each of the actions specified.
- The time required for each of the actions should be specified. These may be *short term* (less than 6 weeks), *medium term* (up to 6 months) and occasionally *long term* (more than 6 months).
- A date for re-auditing the standard, ongoing audit and review should then be set.
- A comparison between the first and second set of audit results will enable the group to evaluate the improvements that have been made and possible areas where further action is required.
- As well as improvements in care the group need to consider the wider effects of involvement in the audit project.

The process of working around the clinical audit cycle is now complete and you will have a good idea of the steps that need to be taken in order to plan a clinical audit project in your area. The first five chapters of this book are summarised in Figure 5.5. This algorithm provides an alternative model with which to think about the stages of a clinical audit project.

Remember that clinical audit is a dynamic process. In theory, there is *no* end to the spiral of activity. However, in practice, problems relating to motivation and the momentum of clinical audit are often encountered. Ongoing support and attention from the wider organisation are required to sustain an effective clinical audit project. This is the subject of Chapters 8 and 9.

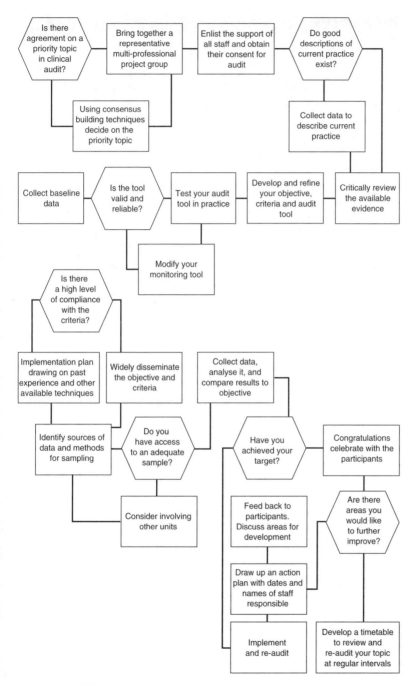

Figure 5.5 **Clinical audit flow chart.**

References

1. ENB 1987 Managing Change in Nurse Education – the process of innovation. ENB, London
2. Lewin K 1951 Field theory in social science. Harper Row, New York
3. Bennis WG, Benne KD, Chin R, Corey KE 1976 The planning of change. Holt Rinehart and Winston, London
4. Johnson G, Scholes K 1993 Exploring corporate strategy, 3rd edn. Prentice Hall, London
5. Senge P 1994 The fifth discipline. Currency Doubleday, New York
6. Rogers EM, Shoemaker F 1971 The communication of innovations. Free Press, New York
7. Lomas J, Enkin M, Anderson GM, Hannah WJ, Vayda E, Singer J 1991 Opinion leaders versus audit and feedback to implement practice guidelines. JAMA 265: 2202–2207
8. Loftus Hills A 1997 The implementation of clinical guidelines. Unpublished teaching material for the Evidence-based Health Care MSc, University of Oxford
9. Walshe K, Spurgeon P 1997 Clinical Audit Assessment Framework, HSMC Handbook series 24. University of Birmingham

6

Variations on a theme

The previous chapters have described criterion-based audit, an approach to clinical audit that is flexible. It allows for the use of different tools and methods whilst following a four stage audit cycle within a framework of continuous improvement. There are other approaches in use throughout the UK which vary in methodology from that already described. A few of these are described below. This is not intended to be an exhaustive list, but attempts to illustrate some of the variations around the theme of clinical audit. The methodologies described in this chapter are:

- benchmarking
- national audit
- care pathways
- TELER system
- peer review.

Benchmarking

Benchmarking is defined as 'the continuous process of measuring products, services, and practices against the toughest competitors or those companies recognised as industry leaders'[1]. It has been widely used in industry and more recently adapted for use in health care in the USA[2,3]. Benchmarking has also been used in the public sector in the UK. It has been suggested that the term best equivalent provider is more appropriate to the public sector than industry leaders[4]. There are four types of benchmark[1]:

1. *Internal benchmarking*: comparing similar processes performed in different parts of the organisation, e.g. admission of in-patients, ordering clinical investigations.
2. *Competitive benchmarking*: comparing the performance of one organisation to that of another on specific measurable

terms, e.g. comparing pressure area care in a centre deemed to be excellent against another similar unit.

3. *Functional benchmarking*: comparison of performance on the same function for all those in a particular sector, e.g. comparing waiting times in accident and emergency departments in every hospital across the UK.

4. *Generic benchmarking*: comparing organisations on a basic practice that is the same regardless of the service provided, e.g. comparing budgets for continuing professional development across professionals in the public sector.

The image most often used to describe benchmarking is that of competition in sport where the current record holder is recognised as the best in their field. Sports people then strive to continually improve their performance to achieve the best in their field. This process is known as benchmarking.

Benchmarking has also been defined as 'the practice of being humble enough to accept that someone else is better at something and being wise enough to learn how to match and even surpass them at it'[5]. From the results of a three year initiative in paediatrics in North West England, benchmarking was found to be a supportive as well as a developmental tool[6]. However, experience in industry suggests that benchmarking is counterproductive for low and medium performing organisations[7] as the exercise can be demoralising.

Essentially, benchmarking involves the same process of defining, implementing, measuring and action planning as described in the previous chapters but audit results are shared across clinical units and organisations with a view to learning from those who do it best.

The process of benchmarking as developed by a network for paediatric benchmarking

Judith Ellis, Senior Lecturer/Practitioner, Preston Acute Hospitals NHS Trust and University of Central Lancashire

Benchmarking involves:

■ agreeing areas of practice where the quality of patient care would benefit from comparison and sharing

- agreeing an overall outcome statement for practice in that area
- agreeing the processes involved in achieving good practice in that area
- identifying and reaching professional consensus on what constitutes best practice – the benchmark (drawing on research, national and local guidelines, customer views and professional consensus)
- compiling a scoring continuum
- using the continuum to score local practice and commenting upon the choice of score
- collating results centrally
- each local unit considering areas for development in the light of their scores
- local units with lower scores using the comments of those with higher scores to plan their developments
- local units with lower scores contacting high scorers for help with change management
- rescoring and comparison with original scores to show development
- best practice statements being periodically reviewed in the light of recent research and developments and the benchmark rescored.

For example, on scoring their benchmark on ethnic sensitivity, practitioners here at Preston recognised that there was a definite need for improvement. The benchmarks were set in conjunction with local consumer groups. Three D/E grade nurses volunteered to take the lead in developing this area of practice with support from F grade team leaders, the lecturer/practitioner and the head of pastoral care at the Trust. The practitioners used regional benchmark results to compare their practice with other units in the region, identifying areas for improvement and the helpful contacts.

It became apparent that in order to meet the needs of the diverse population in Preston, networking across the North West of England would be needed. Benchmarking group members identified particular expertise with certain ethnic groups; for example, staff from Blackburn were able to offer guidance on meeting the needs of the Pakistani community whilst staff from Manchester had experience of working with the Orthodox Jewish community.

The regional benchmarking meeting provided the opportunity for our staff to share their progress and receive encouragement in further developing their action plan. They returned with ideas on accessing interpreter information from computerised personnel records, examples of written information, leaflets, diet sheets and offers of information audio cassettes and video tapes in different languages.

Through openness and sharing of information, practice has developed with minimal repetition of effort. Involvement in benchmarking has helped us develop care for a range of ethnic groups, which would have been very difficult without the regional contacts. By sharing each other's expertise, trigger questions for negotiation of ethnic sensitive care have been developed for all client groups which has been particularly valuable as we attempt to meet the needs of minority ethnic groups rarely cared for in the Trust.

National clinical audit

For some time now, Medical Royal Colleges and professional bodies have been coordinating national clinical audit projects. You may have been involved in collecting data for a national or regional audit project. These projects provide a valuable opportunity to share best practice across organisations with a view to improving standards of care nationally.

In the past, much national audit activity has taken the form of confidential enquiries such as the National Confidential Enquiry into Perioperative Deaths (NCEPOD) and the Confidential Enquiry into Stillbirths and Deaths in Infancy (CESDI). For these sensitive issues it is felt that a confidential enquiry approach will strengthen the information base.

Increasingly, national audits are encouraging clinical teams to share their results more openly similar to the benchmarking model, in order to learn from those achieving good results. Some national audit projects are funded from within the professional organisations themselves. Increasingly they are funded from the Department of Health, and are coordinated by two or more professional bodies working collaboratively.

The NHS Executive in England[8] have set out the purpose of national clinical audit as to:

- encourage and support local providers in further developing the role of clinical audit as a tool for improving the quality of care
- help local providers identify the standards of care they are

achieving compared with national, evidence-based criteria

- demonstrate multidisciplinary and cross-sectoral audit methods which local providers can use for re-audit and adapt for local audit projects
- further develop the use of clinical audit as a crucial tool to enable appropriate change in clinical practice and thereby improve the quality of care
- enable professional bodies to support clinicians locally in maintaining and improving standards of clinical care.

A range of strategies have been employed to collect and collate data from across the country; these include:

- data collection by staff employed by the project travelling to sites to complete audit tools from records at the request of the local medical consultant, arranged by audit staff, e.g. Royal College of Paediatrics and Child Health, Urinary Tract Infection Audit
- data collection by local clinical audit staff using audit tools developed and supplied by the national project, e.g. Royal College of Ophthalmologists working with the Royal College of Nursing and the College of Optometrists on a national audit of cataract surgery.

The National Cataract Audit

The National Cataract Audit is a collation of individual local audits performed in a standardised manner. The project team provided audit tools that included a manual, data collection forms and a database. The manual was designed for non-clinical staff to collect clinical data for the audit under supervision by clinical staff and is intended as a step-by-step guide and reference for the conduct of the audit and it also contained the standards for the audit.

The database allows each centre to hold and keep its audit data locally, with a copy being sent to us for the national database. The database provided a descriptive reporting facility that analyses and prints out the local audit results at the end of the audit. These results are then provided in a format for direct comparison with the standards set at the start.

Personal experiences of participating in the National Cataract Audit at Westbourne Eye Hospital

Liz Hinwood, Clinical Audit Facilitator at the Royal Bournemouth and Christchurch Hospitals NHS Trust

Taking part in the National Cataract Audit was a useful and enlightening experience. Although we have not yet got the formal results, already significant issues have been highlighted. It was important initially to spend time on preparation and to have a named facilitator to lead the audit, to make sure everyone is aware of their role and in agreement to participate before data collection takes place.

The audit has made everyone more aware of documentation. Aspects of care were documented in the theatre ledgers, but not in patient's notes. These included: (a) type of local anaesthetic used, (b) who gave the anaesthetic, whether it was an anaesthetist or ophthalmologist, and (c) type of incision used during the operation. We now have more information on patients meeting the criteria for day case surgery and we know the percentage of patients who have to stay overnight and the reasons for this.

Once a patient is discharged following surgery, the hospital has no feedback on the final visual acuity. The project will give us this information so that we know the number of follow-up visits each patient makes, and the complication rate. The audit has also enabled us to highlight any predisposing medical condition that affects surgery and recovery rate. Information is also available about the percentage of patients who require laser treatment following surgery and the percentage of patients who will need sutures cut or removed in the 3 month period following surgery.

There have, however, been some problems. Some consultants are unhappy about being individually identified on the audit forms, although the facilitator reassured them on several occasions that only she knew their identity on the National Database. Since they were identified by single number, some consultants were still not happy.

On discharge from hospital care, many patients were not given the necessary form to take to the optician, so no final outcome was recorded. Many extra hours were spent contacting patients, and then their optician for their final visual acuity.

All in all it has been a very useful experience even before we have formal results of the audit. We have already identified areas where it will be helpful to carry on collecting information to improve our effectiveness.

Care pathways

Care pathways are described as amalgamating 'all the antici-pated elements of care and treatment of all members of the multidisciplinary team, for a patient or client of a particular case type or grouping within an agreed time-frame, for the achievement of agreed outcomes. Any deviation from the plan is documented as a variance; the analysis of which provides information for the review of current practice.'[9] In essence, this appears very similar to a standard, but a care pathway follows the patient's journey through a number of clinical interventions rather than focusing on one, which clinical audit more com-monly does.

An analysis of the literature describing the use of care path-ways in the USA, Australia and the UK identified a number of steps for their successful development and implementation[10]. These included leadership, education and facilitation. The major benefit reported was the streamlining of patient docu-mentation which will then make collection of data for specific clinical audit projects easier.

As mentioned, variance analysis provides continuous data on whether care is being delivered as set out on the pathway, an in-built clinical audit tool[11]. Analysis of variance data shows up patterns and problems with particular aspects of care delivery which might in turn become a topic for a clinical audit project.

Integrated care pathways – experience of implemen-tation in mental health settings

Maria Harrington, Clinical Audit and Research & Development Manager, Hounslow & Spelthorne Community & Mental Health NHS Trust; Justine Faulkner, Nurse Consultant, Hounslow & Spelthorne Community & Mental Health NHS Trust

In what now seems like the grey and distant mists of time, we jumped aboard the Integrated Care Pathways/Anticipated Recovery Pathways/Pathways in general – bandwagon. The answer to all our prayers/problems? Things have changed but whether or not this is due to an Integrated Care Pathway (ICP) or the term we employed, 'path-way', is open to debate. Our first main area of practice to turn into a pathway was acute adult in-patient care on two sites containing five wards. We duly gathered together our multidisciplinary team of doctors, nurses and therapists (bribed with coffee and cakes) and set forth with our flipchart paper and pens to track care. Several weeks and many sheets of flipchart paper later we had cracked it! A pathway for in-patient care based on current practice was nicely compressed onto three sides of A4 paper containing 76 items or steps on the pathway. This succeeded and failed simultaneously. The successes came from our thinking about how care was delivered and supported by such things as case notes and ward books. New multidisciplinary notes were introduced encompassing Multidisciplinary Team (MDT) progress sheets and care plans. Obscure documents that were historically completed were binned and data collection by numerous professionals reduced. A new culture was emerging and although fraught with practical difficulties like who would write in the notes during a ward round, the two pilot teams battled on. The failure was the pathway itself. It was not completed or followed and was seen as yet another draconian document implemented to 'watch over' practice. We had also in many respects failed to challenge practice; we couldn't, for example, produce evidence from randomised controlled trials (RCTs) for each of the pathway steps, which simply reflected what had taken place historically.

It was time to move on and re-launch. A 'back to the drawing board' approach was taken and we revisited the principles on which the original work had taken place. We had addressed the 'other' agendas such as MDT notes, but had failed to put in place a tool which we could really believe was capable of helping us to monitor the quality of care that was provided to our service users. It is perhaps reflective of the process we used that only now are service users mentioned in this narrative.

Two short-term groups were set up, one containing the multidisciplinary team, the second a group of service users who had a history of in-patient admissions. The service user group looked at our pathway with disbelief – this was not their experience of in-patient care and certainly the key components that they expected were not included. A new pathway began to emerge which was dramatically reduced in terms of quantity and content. The key quality indicators were devised by the service users, e.g. to be offered a cup of tea when being admitted rather than dictatorial instructions to team members to write patients' names on a large dry wipe board. Other changes were suggested such as appointments for ward rounds so patients didn't have to wait around for hours to be seen. Each of the thoughts, ideas and changes were shared between the groups by the facilitators throughout a series of meetings. Changes took place and the new shorter pathway was introduced.

The key question is where are we now? The pathway is there and used to a greater extent than previously, but is by no means perfect. Would we have got where we are without the pathway? Probably, but perhaps not so quickly. Was it useful? Upon reflection, I would say it acted as a change agent but there are numerous change management techniques we could have utilised to attain the same results. At the end of the day, it is a framework, but with momentum gathering on the Clinical Effectiveness Express, pathways may just have found their niche in the world of practice review and development. If each step of the pathway is evidence-based, then their usefulness may be confirmed.

The TELER method

This is a method for making and using clinical notes which requires clinical staff to use a scale to describe the achievement of treatment or care objectives. TELER[12] claims to facilitate clinical audit in the same way as care pathways by simplifying the recording of care and making information accessible. The system has been most widely used within the therapy professions and in rehabilitation settings.

The system allows individual, collaborative, functional and attainable goals to be set and progress towards those recorded using performance indicators. These are scored daily by clinicians with audit taking place at predetermined intervals. TELER is seen to fit with a structure – process – outcome model by providing information on the structure that provides a care programme, the process of that care programme and variables which occur during the episode of care being evaluated. TELER provides this information within one documentation system in a form that displays it clearly for clinical audit purposes[13].

Peer review

There are times when you may wish to review practice in a quicker and simpler way than using a large multi-professional project. There are a number of peer review activities which complement clinical audit, including:

- case review
- clinical supervision
- critical incident analysis.

Case review

Across the UK case review is undertaken in a number of different ways. It can be done concurrently, for example case conferences and ward rounds, so that the practice under review is still unfolding. Alternatively, case review can be conducted with the benefit of hindsight where a case is presented for comment after the care episode is complete.

These are usually multi-professional meetings though often medically dominated. There is tremendous value in inviting the wider team and peer group to share their ideas and experiences. These can also be good forums for bringing in research findings for appraisal and discussion by the group. To maximise their potential for learning everyone's contribution needs to be valued. The introduction of a skilled facilitator may be useful in achieving this.

Suggestions for developing practice often come out of case review discussions without being followed up. A mechanism for systematic action planning, as described in Chapter 5, would stop good ideas getting lost.

Clinical supervision

'This is a term used to describe a formal process of professional support and learning which enables individual practitioners to develop knowledge and competence, assume responsibility for their own practice and enhance consumer protection and safety of care in complex situations. It is central to the process of learning and to the expansion of the scope of practice and should be seen as a means of encouraging self-assessment and analytic and reflective skills.[14]'

It has been increasingly recognised that all health professionals need to continue developing their skills and knowledge throughout their careers. Continuing education and supervision are structured slightly differently between the professional groups, but all have the potential to form complementary relationships with clinical audit.

Individuals' concerns about the way in which they were being asked to make changes as a result of a clinical audit project might become the subject of their clinical supervision meeting. Their journey through the process of integrating evidence into practice might also be written up for inclusion in their professional portfolio. Clinical supervision would be an appropriate forum to address individual problems with any aspect of the clinical audit process, giving practitioners the opportunity to receive support over difficulties they are encountering.

The analytic and reflective skills learned in supervision are the core skills of clinical audit. These abilities to step back and analyse a situation, to reflect on practice as an individual and within a group are transferable to the multi-professional clinical audit group.

Critical incident analysis

Critical incident analysis was first described in the 1950s[15]. It is similar to case review but it usually focuses on one particular aspect of practice which has caused concern rather than a clinical case.

To be effective this multi-professional meeting needs to take place within a non-threatening, no blame, confidential setting. Practitioners must feel able to be honest about the practice under review without fear of criticism or reprisals. The support of an external facilitator is helpful. A critical incident analysis provides an excellent opportunity to look in depth at a particular event and draw out the lessons to be learned. It is a particularly valuable opportunity for team learning where the team can reflect upon the way in which they function together. Just as with the case review, the ideas for improvement are not always acted upon. A clear action plan needs to be devised and implemented. The development of a clinical audit project may well be the result of a critical incident analysis.

Creating the links

All the systems described need to be clearly and carefully linked to clinical audit. In many organisations these various activities all happen but in isolation from one another. Systematic documentation and action planning will help to capture the important issues raised by peer review methods, but these will not realise their potential for practice development unless they take place within an organisational culture which values the contributions made by all staff and encourages change.

Consider the various activities in place within your organisation which are used to develop practice or practitioners. How do they relate to one another and how could this be improved?

 This theme of integration is continued in the following chapters where we will examine the features of a successful clinical audit programme within an organisation.

Summary

- There are a number of useful tools for improving health care quality of which criterion-based audit is only one.
- Benchmarking and national sentinel audits enable practitioners to compare practice across organisations and learn from those achieving excellence.
- Care pathways and the TELER system provide useful mechanisms for planning and documenting care so that outcomes can be readily used for clinical audit.
- Peer review mechanisms complement clinical audit by focusing on specific practice episodes allowing detailed problem-solving and action planning.
- Integration of these activities is necessary if their full potential for enhancing the development of clinical practice is to be realised.

References

1. Camp RC 1989 Benchmarking – the search for industry best practices that lead to superior performance. Quality Press, Milwaukee, WI
2. Campbell AB 1994 Benchmarking: a performance intervention tool. Joint Commission Journal on Quality Improvement 20(5): 225–228
3. Camp RC, Tweet AG 1994 Benchmarking applied to health care. Joint Commission Journal on Quality Improvement 20(5): 229–238
4. Morgan C, Murgatroyd S 1994 Total quality management in the public sector. Open University Press, Buckingham
5. Ellis J 1995 Using benchmarking to improve practice. Nursing Standard 9(35): 25-27
6. Ellis J, Morris A 1997 Paediatric benchmarking: a review of its development. Nursing Standard 12(2): 43–46
7. Ernst & Young 1992 Best practices report: an analysis of management practices that impact performance. Cited in Morgan C, Murgatroyd S 1994 Total quality management in the public sector. Open University Press, Buckingham, p161
8. NHS Executive 1997 Correspondence from the Health Services Division on commissioning national clinical audit projects
9. Johnson S 1997 Pathways of care. Blackwell Science, Oxford
10. Currie L, Harvey G 1997 The origins and use of care pathways in the USA, Australia and the United Kingdom, report no. 15. RCN Institute, Oxford
11. Cheater F 1996 Care pathways: tools for clinical audit? Audit Trends 4: 73–75
12. Le Roux AA 1993 Teler: the concept. Physiotherapy 79(11): 755–758
13. Mawson SJ, McCreadie M 1993 Teler: the way forward in clinical audit. Physiotherapy 79(11): 758–761
14. NHS Management Executive 1993 Vision for the future. Department of Health, London
15. Flanagan JC 1954 The critical incident technique. Psychological Bulletin 1: 327–358

7

Wider considerations

The last three chapters of the book focus on the context of clinical audit, both within an organisation and nationally. This chapter begins by looking at ethical issues, and moves on to discuss the role of the service user or consumer in clinical audit and multi-professional teamwork. The next chapter looks at the organisational support, in particular, facilitation, the importance of strategy, the systems and structures needed to sustain a clinical audit programme and the role of the commissioner in clinical audit. Chapter 9 concludes by exploring clinical audit in the context of health care quality, clinical effectiveness, research and education.

Clinical audit and ethical issues

Over the years, as clinical audit activity has increased, there have been growing concerns that clinical audit projects were not subject to the same process of ethical approval as research projects. In some quarters there were accusations that patients were being overburdened with questionnaires – some of dubious value. The same ethical principles common to any other sphere of clinical practice or research should be applied to clinical audit: autonomy; justice; beneficence – doing good; non-maleficence – doing no harm. There are, however, several specific areas of concern and these include:*

- confidentiality
- consent
- effectiveness of audit
- accountability.

---

* *This section is adapted from a working paper prepared for the NHSE by a group, chaired by Debra Humphris, convened in 1995, by the Clinical Audit Sub Group of the Clinical Outcomes Group.*

Confidentiality

Data collected for audit purposes must protect the identity of patients and clinical staff involved. Patients, clients or their carers must not be identifiable by name, initial, hospital number, bed space number or any other means which would compromise the anonymity of the individual. A European Community directive on data protection permits the use of data for statistical or scientific purposes so long as privacy is safeguarded[1].

Where possible, data should be aggregated so that the performance of an individual staff member is not reported to the wider clinical team. Sometimes it is difficult to disguise the identity of members of clinical staff, particularly when they are the only 'nurse specialist', 'physiotherapist' or 'medical registrar' involved in the audit. Data should therefore be further anonymised to maintain confidentiality and the individuals concerned need to be consulted if information is made available to external bodies. As the results of clinical audit are disseminated widely within an organisation and externally, confidentiality for patients and staff is particularly important.

Consent

It is acceptable practice not to ask for direct patient consent to review records for audit. It is expected that a policy of reviewing material for audit is explicitly mentioned in general information given to patients about the hospital, ward, department, health centre or clinic so that patients are given an opportunity to opt out if they wish. For example:

> The staff of the Birch Centre are actively involved in developing the standards of care that we are able to offer. As a part of this process we value your comments and suggestions. From time to time patient records are reviewed and direct care is observed, to monitor whether or not the standards we set are reached. All information is collected in such a way that patient identity is protected. You may also be asked if you would be willing to fill in a questionnaire or answer some questions about the care that you have received. This is entirely optional and you may feel that you do not wish to participate. This process of setting standards, monitoring and changing practice to improve care is often referred to as clinical audit. If you would like to know more please speak to a member of staff.

If data collection involves questionnaire or interview it is expected that verbal consent will be sought at the time, in a way that puts no pressure on the individual and makes clear that care will not be compromised by refusal to take part. A code of conduct for data collection by questionnaire or interview can be found in Appendix 1.

The consent of all professional staff involved in the processes under review must be sought. As you implement agreed standards of practice all staff involved in the area under review will be made aware of the project and this is an appropriate time to ask for consent for audit.

It is important that before embarking on a project you have considered what course of action you will take if poor practice by an individual staff member is highlighted. It is usual for this to be addressed by the manager of the member of staff concerned, in confidence and as a part of the normal supervision and professional development process. These issues need to be carefully considered and agreed by all staff affected before data collection begins. This is an integral part of gaining staff consent.

The effectiveness of audit

Clinical audit activity represents considerable investment of resources in terms of professional time, not to mention administrative or information systems support. It is therefore important that these resources are used responsibly, that standards are based on good evidence, that the topic under review is a priority, and that staff have the necessary knowledge and skills. Clinical audit whose methodology is poor could be considered unethical in terms of the staff time that is being absorbed. Ethical questions are also raised by changing practice on the basis of inadequate data.

Accountability

If audit results suggest that practice needs improving there is an ethical obligation on the individual practitioners and the unit manager to see that the action plan is implemented. Nurses are expected to 'maintain and improve professional knowledge and competence'[2] as a part of ongoing registration and there is a similar expectation on other clinical professionals.

There is also an accountability to patients/clients which needs consideration. Within each organisation audit activity must be coordinated alongside other initiatives, patient satisfaction surveys and research projects, such that individuals are not expected to fill in more than one questionnaire per visit.

Code of good practice

Within your organisation you need to consider how ethical issues in clinical audit can be addressed for every project undertaken. There has been an increasing interest in ensuring good standards of practice in clinical audit and several Trusts have produced their own codes of conduct or good practice[3].

This may well be something that your local clinical audit committee has considered. A code of conduct provides guidance for those involved in projects to ensure that ethical issues are considered.

Review a local audit report
—How were the ethical issues addressed?
—Are there ethical issues which you would consider inadequately addressed?
—How might you improve any deficits?

Summary

- When designing a clinical audit project ethical issues must be carefully considered. These include *consent, confidentiality, effectiveness of audit* and *accountability*.
- Locally a code of conduct and mechanism to consider ethical issues raised by clinical audit projects should exist.

Consumer involvement

In this section the term consumer has been used to mean patients and their advocates, though there is a clear distinction and there will be times when the two need to be considered separately. Since its inception it has been proposed that clinical audit is informed by the views of patients and clients, but mechanisms for this have not been explicitly discussed. The involvement of patients in clinical audit seems to be considered a good thing but there is little evidence of it in practice. A recent review of the use of the Dynamic Standard Setting System[4] showed that although all those involved claimed that their standards were patient centred and involved patients by asking them for feedback during the measurement phase, only a few had moved beyond this superficial consultation to a model of genuine participation. In 1994 the Department of Health[5] stated:

> Patients and their advocates can influence all stages of the audit process – from standard setting to audit design to drawing up recommendations after analysis. Organisations need to develop mechanisms to ensure that this develops successfully.

Interestingly, the steps of the clinical audit cycle not explicitly mentioned above are topic selection and discussion of results. These areas have been highlighted as needing further development in terms of explicitly involving consumers[6,7]. They are perhaps the most controversial areas. Topic selection involves careful negotiation, balancing the views of professionals, purchasers and consumers. If prioritising topics follows clear criteria, such as those set out in Chapter 2, the process then becomes explicit and open with room for discussion of the various perspectives.

Discussion of clinical audit data is potentially more difficult. It has been suggested in Chapter 4 that consumers may be involved in data collection and therefore in feedback and discussion. This assumes a culture of trust and openness where the ground rules for confidentiality are set out. It also requires that the role of clinical audit is clearly defined and complementary to other professional development activities.

Methods for involving consumers

Increasingly, methods for incorporating patient views are being discussed in the clinical audit literature. Patient satisfaction surveys have been widely used over the past few years both as a means of collecting data to measure against standards and as a way of identifying patient concerns that then inform the selection of topics for clinical audit. The validity of satisfaction as a concept is increasingly being questioned[8]. Patient satisfaction surveys need expert construction. It has been suggested that if the satisfaction of patients is to be maximised then it is necessary to recognise explicitly the decision-making contexts in which the results of patient satisfaction surveys will be used.[9]

Many alternative methods to tap patient experience have been explored. A range of qualitative techniques are particularly useful in clinical audit, such as Critical Incident Technique, consensus conferences, consumer audit[10-12]. Focus groups, in particular, are becoming popular in clinical audit projects.

Using focus groups in clinical audit

Focus groups have been widely used in market research and more recently as a method within the social sciences. 'The purpose of the focus group discussion is to provide a comfortable, and non-threatening situation where individuals with a particular experience in common can discuss their views, feelings, beliefs or opinions, so that these can be recorded and used to inform future practice[13].'

On a practical level – participants should not know one another. The group should be made up of those with a similar experience, e.g. those with a similar illness, carers, older people, children, parents. It is worth holding a number of groups to ensure that views are representative. It is recommended that groups are of between four to twelve people, but seven is considered ideal. Questions should be carefully prepared going from the general to the specific. The person conducting the group should be a skilled facilitator (see Chapter 8). Data are collected by an appointed person taking notes and tape recorded as a back-up[14,15]. Information on qualitative data analysis can be found in Chapter 4.

Using patients' stories

Patients' stories have been used to inform the agenda for quality improvement or clinical audit[16]. Patients were asked to share their experiences of being in hospital and their stories gave detailed accounts of what, to professionals, were considered quality of care issues. These accounts were used as a vehicle for planning service improvement.

Finding appropriate people to participate

It is worth considering carefully how to establish a good input from consumers to your clinical audit project. It is relatively easy to approach current users of a service but there is a wide range of others who could be involved; past patients, potential patients, and carers, also groups representing users, carers and potential patients. The generic nature of the term consumer could lead to differences or even conflicts of views and interests between different groups[7]. In addition, some individuals and groups will be more vociferous and articulate and may be more successful in getting their voices heard.

When selecting consumers for your clinical audit project you need to identify whether you are looking for representation from individuals or from a group. It may be that different representatives are needed for the different stages of the clinical audit cycle. Equally the clinical audit group may benefit from building up a relationship with the same people throughout the project.

Organisational infrastructure

In order for consumers to be involved in clinical audit the necessary structure and mechanisms must exist. The checklist in

---

Box 7.1   Checklist for involving consumers in clinical audit (based on Kelson[7])

Access	Physical access, ramps, doorways etc
	Information on location, timing and transport
	Reimbursement of travelling expenses
	Language, culture and lifestyle issues addressed
Preparation	Training on clinical audit, purpose and methods
	Ensure that participants understand their role and that of others in the group
	Ensure that participants know how to contribute to the group
	Inform participants of the time commitment necessary
	Give participants choices about the way in which they wish to contribute
	Provide training for staff in working in groups with users
Support	Conduct work in an informal group rather than a formal committee
	Ensure participants have a link member whom they can approach with queries or problems
	Ensure that there is always more than one user representative
	Ensure that written materials are all in plain language
	Use the skills of a trained facilitator to help the group dynamics

Box 7.1 may be useful in planning to involve consumers in your clinical audit programme.

It is apparent that if involving consumers is to be taken seriously a significant investment must be made in systems and infrastructure[17]. In addition, the importance of trust and openness cannot be over-emphasised if the consumer contribution is to be taken seriously. This applies equally to successful multi-professional teamwork.

This section has focused on involving consumers in clinical audit projects. Within an organisation an overview of consumer involvement in quality needs to be taken. There needs to be input at a strategic level, planning and prioritising the work of the Trust in this area. This may come from the local Community Health Council or other local representative body. In addition, there needs to be consumer involvement at an organisational level, shaping the ideas of the clinical audit team, and involvement in training programmes on clinical audit.

Below is an example of the role of a consumer representative within a national clinical guidelines project from the Royal College of Psychiatrists.

Involving service users in developing clinical practice guidelines

Claire Palmer, Royal College of Psychiatrists' Research Unit

Background

The Royal College of Psychiatrists' Research Unit published its first clinical practice guideline in March 1998. This is the first guideline produced by the College Research Unit (CRU) Clinical Practice Guidelines (CPG) Programme. A fundamental value of the CRU is to involve service users in our work wherever possible. It was therefore important for service users to be involved in the development of our first CPG 'The Management of Imminent Violence: a clinical practice guideline to support mental health services'.

Why involve service users?

The CPG Programme believes that it is important to involve service users for the following reasons:

- they are experts about their illness, disability or condition
- they have in-depth knowledge and experience of health services
- they are directly affected by the content of the guideline
- they are potential guideline users and can assist in their implementation
- their views and experiences are currently under-represented in the literature, particularly research literature, so alternative methods to obtain service users' views need to be found
- both the CRU and mental health service user organisations believe that service users should always have the opportunity to be active participants in (rather than passive recipients of) care and therefore in the development of clinical practice guidelines.

The benefits of involving service users include the production of more useful, accurate, credible and appropriate guidelines.

Guidance for involving service users

A seminar on involving service users in clinical guidelines was organised in May 1995 by the Royal College of Nursing in collaboration with the Patients' Association, the College of Health, the Royal College of Psychiatrists, the Royal College of General Practitioners, the British Psychological Society and the Lancashire College of Nursing. The audience, comprising guideline developers and service user organisations, was asked to produce guidance on involving users in guideline development[18]. From this we drew up guidance for our CPG Programme:

- service users should be involved in all development levels, from topic selection to guideline dissemination and implementation
- service users should be collaborators in the process, rather than just consulted
- service users, like everyone else, should be paid for the time they spend working on guideline development
- more than one service user should be involved where possible
- the same criteria should be used for selecting service users and professionals (for example, ability to do the job in hand, ability to work well in a small multidisciplinary group etc.).

How were service users involved?

Service users were involved in every stage of the guideline development process. A sample of 100 service users, and 26 voluntary sector organisations, were asked to contribute to the selection of the topic of the first guideline (the management of violence was in the top five priorities selected by all groups surveyed, including service users, out of a choice of 56 topics). Two service user representatives are members of the CPG Steering Group and one service user is a member of the work group established to develop the CRU's first guideline (the CPG work groups have less than eight members so are not able to have more than one representative). Service users were given the opportunity to participate in the systematic review which forms the cornerstone of guideline development, although this was not taken up for our first guideline.

The work group service user representative led a User and Carer Consultation Group in developing a two-stage process for obtaining the views and experiences of service users. Firstly, the major user organisations in the UK were sent a questionnaire asking for their views on the six topic areas covered by the systematic review. In addition, the UK Advocacy Network was commissioned to organise and provide facilitators for three focus groups of service users with experience of different types of mental health services (secure units, acute units and community services) on our behalf. Service users were asked to make recommendations to the work group in the six areas covered by the systematic review. This information was incorporated into the final guideline statements and a summary of the focus group discussions included as an appendix to the guideline report.

Finally, voluntary sector organisations were involved in the extensive external review of the guideline and in its dissemination.

Being a service user representative

Nina Rideout, Service User Representative, CPG Work Group

Selection of service users

It is important to select someone with 'appropriate' experience of being a service user, i.e. someone who has *direct*, and preferably recent, experience of the illness, condition, disability or services of interest. If possible, select someone who has some experience of working with committees and/or work groups, or provide them with appropriate training and support. It is an advantage to select someone who has some clinical knowledge of the field of interest and is reasonably familiar with the medical terms and drug names used. Finally, it is important to select someone who has an overview of the views of other users and who understands the diversity of views and the needs of different users. National and local user groups can be tremendously helpful in identifying and recommending the right person.

The following issues need to be taken into account by health workers:

- service users can be ill (this sounds obvious but careful consideration should be given to how the needs of both the service user and the work group can be met)
- health workers may need to clarify clinical or methodological issues
- other work group members need to be willing and able to work alongside service users as equal team members
- work groups need to be prepared to put extra effort into recruiting and supporting service users.

The following are things that help service users to be an active work group member:

- good administrative support, e.g. comprehensive, jargon-free minutes
- a work group that operates as a team
- really being and feeling involved
- making meetings informal, sociable and fun.

I enjoyed being a member of the CPG work group and felt involved as an equal. Being on a work group and developing the CPG was a learning experience and has boosted my confidence.

Draw up a list of barriers to consumer involvement in your workplace and for each barrier propose solutions.

Summary

- It is important to involve consumers at all stages of the clinical audit cycle.
- A variety of methods exist to involve consumers, including focus groups, and involvement on clinical audit committees
- It is important to consider how a range of good consumer input can be established.
- The necessary access, preparation and support must be provided.

The place of uni-professional clinical audit

You will remember from Chapter 2, when selecting a topic for clinical audit, all the relevant professional groups are consulted and involved in the project. Just occasionally a priority topic emerges which only affects one professional group. This may be an aspect of a bigger project.

There remains a place for uni-professional clinical audit, but the same guidance applies to the development of the project. Even if the aspect of care under review only concerns one group, the rest of the organisation will still be affected and therefore information on the progress of the project should be widely disseminated. Below is an example of a good uni-professional audit project.

Infection control and patient washbowls: staff understanding of best practice

Michele Grange and Christina Maslen, Royal National Hospital for Rheumatic Diseases (RNHRD) NHS Trust, Bath

Background

This audit was conducted amongst nursing staff of all grades in one ward of the Rheumatology Unit at the RNHRD, Bath. It arose as a result of concerns by the nursing sister that there was a problem associated with staff handling of patient washbowls.

Problem

Anecdotal evidence of:

- poor practice relating to handling and storage of patient washbowls
- lack of understanding of best practice

leading to potential risk to patients of cross infection.

Audit objectives

- To determine whether nursing staff deal with washbowls effectively.
- To determine whether nursing staff understand the rationale behind the correct procedures for dealing with patient washbowls.

What is best practice – where is the evidence?

■ Literature review
■ RNHRD NHS Trust Infection Control Policy and Procedure Manual

Audit indicators and data collection

Using the evidence, indicators were developed which reflected the issues to be addressed. Self-administered questionnaires were used to collect data on practice and knowledge.

Audit criteria and results

Criteria	Expected	Results
1. Nurses to state that washbowls to be cleaned:		
a. with detergent and water	100%	83%
b. rinsed after cleaning	100%	92%
2. Nurses to state that, after cleaning, washbowls to be dried either physically or upside down in air	100%	100%
3. Nurses to identify appropriate storage of washbowls	100%	50%
4. Nurses to be aware of conditions likely to encourage bacterial growth in washbowls	100%	67%
5. Nurses to have attended infection control training session in last 12 months	100%	8%
6. Nurses to be aware of existence of Trust policy on cleaning washbowls	100%	25%
7. Nursing staff to feel knowledgeable about infection control issues	100%	50%

Action taken

The results indicated that any necessary action needed to be focused on providing education and training.

A training session, attended by all nurses, was held covering:

■ appropriate cleaning of washbowls
■ appropriate storage of washbowls
■ conditions promoting bacterial growth
■ reminder of Trust Infection Control Policy and Procedure Manual – and where it can be found for reference.

Re-audit

After 4 weeks, nurses were then observed handling washbowls on the ward over a 2 week period.

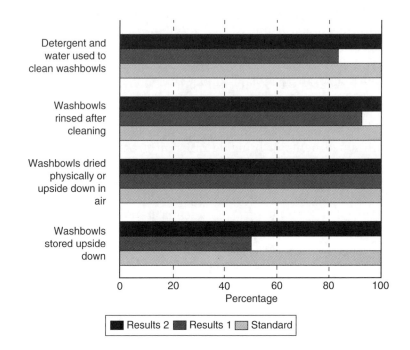

Figure 7.1 **Nurses' handling of patient washbowls – improvement**

Outcome – changes in practice

- Regular teaching sessions on infection control are now to be held every 3 months.
- Current developments in research in infection control are to be put on the staff notice board.
- A 'bug poster' has been put up in the sluice as a reminder to staff.
- Staff questionnaires will be used to evaluate the content and efficacy of training sessions.

This audit project not only improved the way nurses handled washbowls, but also raised staff awareness and understanding of infection control issues in general.

Multi-professional teamwork

Increasingly, it is expected that clinical audit will be multi-professional and multi-agency (across organisational boundaries) to reflect the patient's experience of care. The development of multi-professional teams is vital to clinical audit[19] if it is genuinely to enhance the quality of care. It has been suggested that the very essence of multi-professional audit is teamwork.[20] As we have seen, there remains a place for uni-professional audit but the vast majority of clinical topics need addressing by a number of professional groups and agencies as very little care is delivered by one professional group in isolation. There can be significant benefits of bringing different groups together for a clinical audit project, notably an increased understanding of the roles and contributions of others and improved communication.

As described in Chapter 2, the clinical audit group provide the leadership for any given clinical audit project. The membership of this group may be quite fluid with a core membership to see the task to completion, and a peripheral group of others who are involved as needed. This group is likely to report to another multi-professional forum, the clinical audit committee or quality steering group whose role is to plan and coordinate activity across an organisation. The clinical audit group is also accountable to the wider multi-professional team involved with the clinical topic under review on whose commitment the success of the project depends. It is clear therefore that bringing together the individuals and groups who make up the health care team, even for one clinical area, is a challenge. In the words of a recent report on primary health care audit[21]:

> Making multi-disciplinary teams work effectively, and managing change constructively will be invariably more testing than mastering the technicalities of the audit process.

Barriers to multi-professional teamwork

Misunderstandings and tribal boundaries between professional groups can hinder the development of collaborative audit. These are often a legacy of the histories of the development of audit in the different professions. Three common misgivings that nurses have about becoming involved in multi-professional audit include[20]:

- the compounding of difficulties found in uni-disciplinary audit
- inter-professional fears
- the wide variety of available quality systems and tools.

Additional barriers to multi-agency projects

- agreeing the funding of the project – who is to pay for what
- difficulties in sharing information across organisations
- differences in organisational culture between organisations/agencies.

There is often a perceived imbalance of power making true teamwork, with mutual respect and equity between professions, difficult to achieve. 'Although all health professionals should have an equal contribution to make choosing the topics for audit, in virtually all cases such topics are chosen by the medically qualified leaders of the service'[22]. It could be suggested that this dominance in decision-making often extends well beyond topic selection to decisions affecting the rest of the clinical audit cycle.

A regional study to assess progress towards multi-professional audit described obstacles to nurses' participation[23]:

- hierarchical nurse and doctor relationships
- lack of commitment from senior doctors and managers
- poor organisational links between departments of quality and audit
- workload pressures and lack of protected time
- availability of practical support
- lack of knowledge and skills.

There are no quick and easy solutions to difficulties of team functioning as many problems are deeply embedded within an organisation's culture. Chapter 5 describes change management strategies which may be useful to help unravel your local situation. A few practical suggestions might include:

- *Joint educational initiatives* – by learning about clinical audit together many of the problems of diverse approaches and methods are addressed as well as the social effect of getting away from the workplace together.
- *Team building half day* – many units already have half a day per month set aside for clinical audit. Invite members of professions who do not normally attend and focus on team building with the help of a skilled facilitator.
- *Forming clinical audit groups* – new project groups need time to build relationships before launching into action. You may wish to consider making the first meeting a meal or social event.

A team quadrant has been described identifying teams in two dimensions: formal or informal; and temporary or permanent (Fig. 7.2)[24]. Clinical audit project groups could be described as temporary and formal as they have the official recognition of the organisation and exist only for the duration of the project. The problem with such teams is that there is often little management commitment to either resourcing their temporary work or acting upon the results of their recommendations.

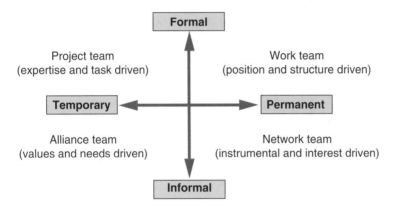

Figure 7.2 **A team quadrant.**

Models of multi-professional/agency clinical audit

A representative clinical audit group of six to eight individuals with a skilled facilitator provides a democratic model of ensuring the involvement of all those affected by the issue under review. However, sometimes the practicalities of getting a group to meet at a time which is acceptable to all means that meetings are just not possible.

It may be that a smaller core working group can be convened who consult nominated representatives regularly to keep them up to date with progress and invite their comments and suggestions. Alternatively, if it is impossible even to convene a small group it may fall to the audit facilitator or project leader to liaise with the various representatives. When differences of opinion arise, ad hoc meetings can then be arranged to discuss specific matters.

Below is an example of a multi-professional interface audit, which actively involves service users.

The patient as the true focus of an interface audit project

Jill Gladstone, Clinical Audit Coordinator, Royal Devon & Exeter NHS Trust

Thyrotoxicosis is a common condition in which there can be problems with both diagnosis and the provision of well controlled, effective treatment. The experiences of a patient led to the development of an interface audit between primary and secondary care in which the patient was a key member of the multi-professional steering committee and actively involved in all stages of the audit. Involvement of the patient and access to his views and suggestions provided valuable insight for clinicians into all aspects of the investigation and management of thyrotoxicosis.

Audit criteria aimed to determine whether:

■ diagnosis of thyrotoxicosis was confirmed by biochemical results
■ medical treatment was continued for the recommended minimum 12 month period
■ biochemical status was regularly monitored
■ referrals to endocrine specialists were seen within one month
■ patients felt sufficiently informed about their condition and its management.

An appropriate sample of patients was identified by the GPs. Clinical management was followed through primary and secondary care and patients' views of the service sought using a written questionnaire which was designed in conjunction with the patient from the steering committee.

The audit demonstrated variations in referrals and clinical management. Delay in diagnosis was a problem for several patients and there was a general need for better information about the condition and its treatment.

Specific outcomes included:

■ presentation by patient representative of findings from the questionnaire at a GP study day and a major clinical education meeting in secondary care
■ production of local guidelines for GPs
■ introduction of an open access thyroid clinic in secondary care
■ improvements in patient information including the provision to patients of graphical print-outs of biochemical results

- improved links and support from secondary care for primary care nurses
- identification of research proposals.

Thinking of your own clinical team identify the factors that will enhance the further development of multi-professional team-work and the factors restraining such development. Then consider how you could strengthen the positive forces and weaken those opposing change. See 'force field analysis' in Chapter 5.

Summary

- Most clinical audit projects are best addressed by a multi-professional team of those involved.
- Barriers to effective teamwork and to working across agencies and sectors exist and require creative solutions.
- Joint educational initiatives provide one way of helping staff come together.
- There are a number of different models of collaborative clinical audit.

References

1. Smith MF 1996 Data protection, health care, and the new European directive. BMJ 312: 197–198
2. UKCC 1992 Code of professional conduct. UKCC, London
3. Ferris M 1996 A code of good practice for the conduct of clinical audit. Network issue 22, pp 1–3
4. Morrell C, Harvey G, Kitson AL 1995 The reality of practitioner based quality improvement, report no. 14. National Institute for Nursing, Oxford
5. Department of Health 1994 The evolution of clinical audit. DoH, London, p 12
6. Rigge M 1994 Involving patients in clinical audit. Quality in Health Care 3(suppl): 52–55
7. Kelson M 1995 Consumer involvement initiatives in clinical audit and outcomes. College of Health, London
8. Williams B 1994 Patient satisfaction: a valid concept? Social Science and Medicine 38(4): 509–516
9. Scott A, Smith RD 1994 Keeping the customer satisfied: issues in the interpretation and use of patient satisfaction surveys. International Journal of Quality in Health Care 6(4): 353–359
10. Powell J, Lovelock R, Bray J, Philp I 1994 Involving consumers in assessing service quality: benefits of using a qualitative approach. Quality in Health Care 3(4): 199–202
11. Dennis N 1995 Consumer audit in the NHS. British Journal of Health Care Management 1(9): 472–474
12. Fitzpatrick R, Bolton M 1994 Qualitative methods for assessing health care. Quality in Health Care 3: 107–113
13. McIver S 1995 Focus groups and discussion groups – are they the same? Journal of the Association of Quality in Healthcare 3(2): 43–48
14. Preston C 1995 All you ever need to know about running focus groups but were too afraid to ask. Audit Trends 3(4): 140–143
15. McIver S 1991 An introduction to obtaining the views of users of health services. King's Fund Centre, London
16. Adair L 1994 The patient's agenda. Nursing Standard 9(9): 20–23
17. Brotchie J, Wann M 1993 The training needs of lay people working in health. The Patients Association, London
18. Duff L et al 1995 Clinical guidelines: involving patients and service users. Royal College of Nursing, London
19. Department of Health 1994 The evolution of clinical audit. DoH, London
20. McKenna H 1995 A multi-professional approach to audit. Nursing Standard 9(46): 32–35
21. Clinical Outcomes Group 1995 Clinical Audit in Primary Health Care. Department of Health, London, p 28
22. Hopkins A 1996 Clinical audit: time for reappraisal? Journal of the Royal College of Physicians 30(5): 415–425
23. Cheater FM, Keane M 1998 Nurses' participation in audit: a regional study. Quality in Health Care 7: 27–36
24. Higgs M, Rowland D 1992 All pigs are equal? Management Education and Development 23(4): 349–362

8
Supporting clinical audit

In order for clinical audit to thrive there needs to be a culture within the organisation where there is a willingness to change – a philosophy of improvement. Clinical audit is a dynamic process and change is integral to the improvement of practice. As often as not change is required throughout the organisation. Changes may be needed in systems or structures in order for clinical staff to practise effectively. There is therefore a central role for change agents, those whose role is to support and enable change. This chapter describes in some detail the change agent role, that of the facilitator in clinical audit, and goes on to describe the systems and structures that need to be in place for a programme of clinical audit to function within an organisation.

Facilitation

To enable the multi-professional group to work together it can be helpful to draw on the skills of a trained facilitator. The term facilitation is used to describe a process of helping, guiding and enabling. In the context of clinical audit, the role of the facilitator is to help the clinical audit group to assimilate the evidence and come to a common understanding of clinical audit methodology, to guide the clinical audit project from planning to reporting and to enable the group to work effectively together to that end. The role is to support the group during the process of working through the clinical audit cycle. This involves paying attention to different types of need. These can be defined as task, group and individual needs[1].

- *Task needs* refer to the clinical audit project itself. In this respect, the facilitator's role is to provide the group with the knowledge and practical support they need to work through the stages of defining the standard, audit and action planning.
- *Group needs* refer to the collective needs of the group. The facilitator's role is to promote team-building and to develop a

level of trust and understanding within the group, so that it can work freely and productively.

- *Individual needs* relate to the needs of individual members within the group. The facilitator's role is to ensure that individuals' needs for security and support within the group are met and that individuals are enabled to participate equally and democratically within the group.

Although distinct, these three needs can be seen to overlap to some extent, as illustrated in Figure 8.1.

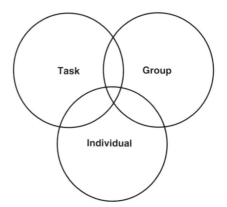

Figure 8.1 Different types of need in clinical audit. (After Adair[1].)

Therefore, if one group of needs is neglected or unfulfilled in any way, this impacts on to the other needs and limits the extent to which they can be met. For example, imagine a group that is very cohesive and where members are supportive both of each other and the collective team. However, despite this high level of support within the group, they fail to focus on achieving the vision or task and drift from one topic of conversation to another during the course of meetings. The long-term effect of failing to address task needs will eventually begin to influence both individual and group experiences (Fig. 8.2). Some team members may become impatient at the apparent lack of progress and display their impatience as irritability during the course of subsequent group meetings; this will affect relationships within the group as a whole.

The facilitator, therefore, has a key role to play in ensuring a healthy balance is maintained between meeting task, group and individual needs during the clinical audit cycle. Hence the role

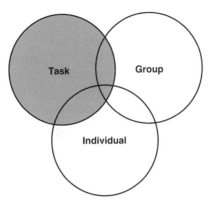

Figure 8.2 **How failure to meet task needs has a knock-on effect on both group and individual needs. (After Adair[1].)**

is one of project manager, educator and harmoniser and requires the following:

- A knowledge of clinical audit, its development in the various professional groups, a detailed understanding of its principles and methods; skills in a variety of educational techniques to enhance small group learning.
- An understanding of project management, the culture and structures within the organisation, and how to tap into the necessary expertise and resources available locally, e.g. library facilities, statistical advice.
- A knowledge of group processes and a range of skills in dealing with complex dynamics and interactions within a small group setting; familiarity with techniques of team building and exercises to enhance team functioning.

It is apparent that the facilitator needs careful preparation for the role and may well require specific training. The facilitator needs to be seen as credible by the clinical audit group and this may mean that they are expected to have a relevant clinical background and a good knowledge of the issue under review as well as possessing the attributes listed above. There are advantages and disadvantages to this.

An 'insider' who is a member of the team for whom they are acting as facilitator may well be the ideal choice, having a full understanding of the peculiarities of the situation and the particular team dynamics. By the same token they could be seen by some team members as partisan and it may be difficult for the individual to remain neutral if he or she has strong views on the topic. It may be more appropriate to use an 'outsider', someone from the audit support team or a member of another clinical team. Not having an intimate involvement with the issue under review may give the outside facilitator the necessary objectivity to deal with problems effectively.

Heron's dimensions and modes of facilitation

One model suggests that the facilitator role involves an ability to operate in six dimensions (Box 8.1)[2].

Box 8.1   Heron's six key dimensions of facilitation
■ planning ■ meaning ■ confronting ■ feeling ■ structuring ■ valuing

These dimensions could be seen linking into the three needs of the group. The *task* needs demand that the facilitator *plans* and *structures* the experience of the group. The clinical audit cycle provides the *structure* for the project and careful *planning* is needed to allow sufficient time for each phase without losing momentum.

The facilitator enables the *group* needs to be met by developing the *meaning* dimension in creating a shared understanding of the purpose, the language and the potential of the project. In addition, the facilitator helps to build up a sense of group identity, increasing the level of trust within the group by being sensitive to concerns and *feelings*.

Individual needs are also the concern of the facilitator who is responsible for ensuring that group members feel *valued* and respected within the group. It is also important that the facilitator addresses problems within the group and is willing to *confront* individuals who are causing difficulty for others.

Styles of facilitator intervention

Within each of the six dimensions listed above, the facilitator can adopt different styles of intervention, depending on the degree of power and control he or she wishes to have over the interaction (Box 8.2). There is no right or wrong way to facilitate a group. Facilitators need to be true to themselves, their individual style and be adaptable to the group needs and the pressures imposed by the organisation.

Box 8.2   Facilitator styles of intervention. (Adapted from Heron[2])

DIRECTIVE   The facilitator is responsible for all decision-making and action within the dimension

COOPERATIVE   The facilitator works collaboratively with the group to make decisions

NON-DIRECTIVE The facilitator devolves all responsibility for decision-making and intervention to the group

---

By combining the six dimensions with the three possible styles of intervention, the facilitator role can be conceptualised within the matrix shown in Box 8.3. This gives an idea of the range of different ways a facilitator might interact with a group. Within any clinical audit project there may be times when the facilitator needs to be very directive and heavily structure the group's experience and other times when he or she sits back and appears to let the group get on with it.

Box 8.3   Modes of operation for the facilitator

	Planning	Meaning	Confronting	Feeling	Structuring	Valuing
Directive						
Cooperative						
Non-directive						

The matrix suggests a possible total of 18 modes of operation for the facilitator. The facilitator should be able to operate in any of the 18 boxes, depending on the needs of the group or individuals within the group at any one time. The skill of the facilitator is being able to adopt the *appropriate* style of facilitation at the *appropriate* time. This requires a range of interpersonal, communication and group skills – skills that are developed through experience and through ongoing reflection and evaluation of the role.

When you are starting as a facilitator it may be useful to co-facilitate, to facilitate a group with a more experienced colleague who can give you support and feedback. Alternatively, you could ask the group for feedback or ask a trusted member of the group to be a critical friend.

Facilitating multi-professional clinical audit or 'how to keep your balloon up without the hot air'

Marian Naidoo, Clinical Development Manager, East Wiltshire Health Care NHS Trust

Life as a clinical audit facilitator can be both challenging and frustrating but it can also be incredibly rewarding. I have worked as a clinical audit facilitator in a Community Trust for five years and during those years have learnt a lot about teamwork and group dynamics. I have also become an expert peace maker and groveller and I am sure my own background in Nursing, Education and Performing Arts is a perfect combination for this role!

Let's face it, a team that comes together to undertake a clinical audit can be working together for the first time. The team can be both multi-professional and multi-agency and can have no more in common than belonging to that team. Despite this, the expectations we have of them are high. They are expected to look critically and objectively at what they do, agree and accept criteria for standards to measure the delivery of care provided by them and then be open to a change in practice if so required. It is not surprising that this process can some-times be a difficult one to facilitate.

The multi-professional clinical audit process itself can be an excel-lent vehicle for developing a team. One of the first multi-professional clinical audits I facilitated came about when a school nurse who had just completed an asthma diploma came to talk to me about her con-cerns regarding young children at school with asthma. We agreed that this would be a good topic for audit and identified a team that includ-ed professionals from both primary and secondary care and from the education service. She was rather nervous about inviting these indi-viduals to work with her. The audit process in this instance enabled those individuals to develop a common understanding of the care process as a whole and from this a mutual respect and a greater understanding of each other's professional roles developed. The benefits to the children following the audit are, I suppose, somewhat predictable but the benefits to the individuals taking part in this audit were also significant. In my experience this was not unusual, but the role of the facilitator in this context was crucial, particularly in a supporting and motivating role and in helping to enable the process of change to take place.

In order to implement a programme of clinical audit across an organisation it is useful to have a network of facilitators to guide the individual projects who are themselves enabled and guided in the role by a key facilitator. These necessary supportive structures are the subject of the next section.

What contribution could a facilitator have made to groups you have been involved with? Who within your organisation could take on the role of facilitator?

Summary

- The role of the facilitator is to enable the clinical audit group to work efficiently, effectively and cohesively together.
- The facilitator should be specifically trained for the role with knowledge of clinical audit, project management and group processes.
- The person chosen for the role may belong to the clinical team concerned with the topic or come from elsewhere.

Sustaining a clinical audit programme

As emphasised in Chapter 1, one of the keys to sustaining clinical audit in practice is to establish a supportive organisational structure from the initial stage of implementation; one which promotes accountability and decision-making at the level of service delivery. Such a structure is developed and maintained by empowering practitioners to take responsibility for their own practice. Within this empowering process, trained facilitators play a vital role, providing practitioners at a local level with the necessary knowledge, skills and support to assume ownership and control of clinical audit.

At the same time, the facilitator should promote open lines of communication in as many directions as possible: from clients to practitioners; from practitioners to managers; from managers to clients; from one group of practitioners to another and so on.

In order to address both the organisational and practitioner requirements during implementation, a multi-level, multi-dimensional framework for clinical audit should be considered. This involves addressing clinical audit at three key levels, described as the *strategic level*, the *organisational level* and the *operational level*.

The strategic level

At this level, it is important that an organisation identifies its philosophy of quality and what is to be achieved by introducing a clinical audit programme. This should be discussed and agreed at a board level, integrating the requirements of legislation, the commissioners and the organisational business plans. This may involve the formation of a quality steering or strategy group to draw together clinical audit with organisational quality, clinical effectiveness and clinical governance. To be successful it must have explicit leadership and support from the chief executive.

The organisational level

At an organisational level, the focus is on developing systems and structures to support the implementation of the clinical audit programme. This covers a range of issues, including education and training, support and networking, communication and feedback of data, indexing and dissemination of information. Coordination of this type of organisational activity is undertaken by someone in a key facilitator role supported by audit staff. Typically this person may be called the clinical audit manager, clinical effectiveness or practice development coordinator.

The clinical level

Having established the strategic and organisational framework, the emphasis is on making quality happen at the clinical level. This is generally undertaken on an individual project basis with clinical audit teams, supported by a local facilitator representing a number of clinical areas according to the project topic.

Box 8.4 summarises key issues for consideration at the strategic, organisational and clinical levels of clinical audit. A vital factor in the success of the clinical audit programme is ensuring that the three levels communicate effectively and are coordinated towards achieving the same goal – the improvement of the quality of care.

Box 8.4   Framework for clinical audit

STRATEGIC LEVEL

Clinical audit committee or quality steering group

Responsible for:
philosophy and ethical framework
aims, objectives and annual planning cycle
links to business planning and contracting process
integration with organisational quality
links with clinical governance and effectiveness

ORGANISATIONAL LEVEL

Clinial effectiveness/ audit team

Responsible for:
education programme
support and facilitation
communication and feedback
computer support and indexing

CLINICAL LEVEL

Clinical audit project groups

Responsible for:
undertaking clinical audit projects
programme of re-audit and review

Maintaining the communication up, down and across these levels can be enhanced by using a facilitation model.

The role of the local facilitator

Local facilitators support clinical audit groups through individual projects. The groups usually exist for the duration of the project and may reconvene occasionally to review their standards in the light of new evidence. The facilitator therefore has an important role to play in ensuring that the group completes the clinical audit cycle. This provides a powerful motivating factor by maintaining momentum and promoting further improvement. The local facilitator also ensures that clinical audit results are fed back into the organisational system, through communication and collaboration with the key facilitator.

Key facilitator

Where the local facilitator focuses primarily on supporting the clinical team, the key facilitator typically functions at an organisational level. The key facilitator's role is therefore more concerned with creating and supporting the overall organisational framework for clinical audit. This involves raising awareness about clinical audit throughout the organisation, establishing training courses for all levels and disciplines of staff and selecting and training facilitators to work with local groups.

In addition to this educational role, the key facilitator also assumes responsibility for coordinating the clinical audit programme, for example through creating a database of projects and by setting up communication and support structures, such as network groups and local newsletters. In many cases, these may also link into national networks such as the Royal College of Nursing's Dynamic Quality Improvement Network. The key facilitator is also responsible for operationalising the strategic integration of clinical audit with other organisational quality initiatives, clinical effectiveness and clinical governance strategies.

Hence, the key facilitator functions very much as a catalyst and agent of change, creating and developing opportunities for quality improvement, and continuously cascading information throughout the organisation. This is certainly a complex role to perform, requiring a range of communication, interpersonal and educational skills and abilities. Ideally, the person taking on this role should be in a full-time, funded support post, with no clinical line management responsibility.

Administrative and IT support

The key facilitator role is usually supported by the clinical audit office. It is here that the necessary administrative systems are set up to classify and index clinical audit projects, to send out reminders that re-audits are due and that standards need reviewing.

There are a number of computer software packages on the market specifically designed for clinical audit both in terms of helping staff work through individual projects and to classify and index them, for example the DQI Toolbox. Many organisations have set up systems using their existing software. Where computer systems are networked indexes of projects and proformas or prompts for project planning are instantly accessible in all clinical areas. Whatever option is chosen, making the most of the available information technology within an organisation can minimise the paperwork generated by clinical audit activity.

Clinical audit committees/quality steering groups

Clinical audit committees provide the strategic overview of clinical audit within an organisation. They are usually responsible for the clinical audit budget, for coordination of reporting on clinical audit activity and for agreeing the annual clinical audit plan with the commissioners. They may be responsible for planning local conferences, prizes, study days and allocating money to individual projects.

As a multi-professional group including consumer representatives and possibly representatives from other agencies they are prone to the same problems of group dynamics as the local clinical audit groups. Your committee may have a very effective chairperson. It can be useful to complement the chairperson's role with a facilitator for the clinical audit committee itself. What follows are two examples of strategic approaches to organising clinical audit and clinical effectiveness, one for a large university teaching hospital and another collaborative approach to clinical audit for community care.

A strategic approach to clinical audit

Susan Lowson, Quality Development Manager, Southampton University Hospital NHS Trust

There is a formalised approach to quality improvement within the Southampton University Hospitals Trust and clear roles and responsibilities for managing it. Quality forms an integral part of both corporate and individual objectives. The Trust Mission Statement defines quality as 'pursuing excellence in everything we do'.

The Director of Nursing and Patient Services is responsible for leading and coordinating the development of the quality improvement programme. The Director is supported by the Quality Development Manager and works closely with the Clinical Effectiveness Team who are managed by the Medical Director (Fig. 8.3).

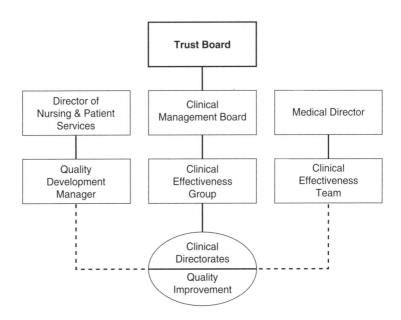

Figure 8.3 **Organisational structure.**

The clinical effectiveness programme is managed by a Clinical Effectiveness Group (CEG) chaired by a consultant accountable through the Medical Director to the Clinical Management Board.

The CEG leads on the promotion of the use of evidence-based practice and raising the profile of clinical effectiveness within the Trust.

The Trust's strategy for clinical effectiveness is to:

■ Ensure that all patients managed in the Trust receive clinical services which:

    a. are delivered on the basis of an integration of research evidence (or on the basis of best (national) clinical practice where not available) and individual clinical expertise

    b. are the best affordable

    c. are as safe as possible in terms of clinical risk.

- Demonstrate excellence in clinical care when this exists.
- Enable the introduction of clinical governance into the Trust.

Responsibility for the delivery of these actions necessary to achieve the objectives rests with the Clinical Effectiveness Group, which is a subcommittee of the Clinical Management Board, working essentially through the Clinical Effectiveness Team but with others such as the Risk Management Group, and the Directors of Research and Development and Medical Education, in order to influence the delivery of clinical care.

The clinical care provided by the Trust must be the best possible care option for the circumstances in which it is given. This divides into three main spheres: inform, change and monitor[3].

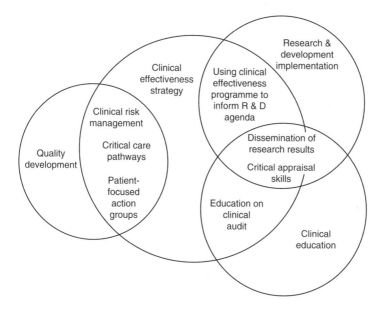

Figure 8.4 Linking research, quality, clinical effectiveness and audit.

Inform

There must be sufficient good evidence on clinical and cost effectiveness which is made available to the NHS in a way which informs clinicians, patients and managers. They will need evidence from research but also information about patterns of care, population needs and the availability of resources[3].

The Clinical Effectiveness Group interprets this as:

- Maintenance and updating of an index of national / local expert clinical guidelines and care pathways.
- Working with the Director of Research and Development to improve the dissemination of results of recent research.
- Working with the Director of Medical Education and clinical tutors to ensure that skills needed to deliver clinically effective care feature on educational programmes for all grades of doctor. This includes critical appraisal skills, accessing computerised information, managing clinical risk and audit methodology.
- Working with directorates to ensure non-medical staff who affect patient care have access to education about critical review of practice, managing clinical risk, accessing computerised information and audit methodology.
- Working with Wessex Medical Library to facilitate access to information for all grades of staff.
- Publicise and consider issues related to national clinical indicators as they become available.

Change

> Local strategies need to encourage those who make decisions to use this information to review and, where necessary, change routine clinical and managerial practice[3].

The process of change will always create tensions amongst staff and needs to be managed sensitively. The Group is pursuing this through:

- Working with Purchasers, particularly the local health authority, to ensure clinically effective purchasing.
- Examining the potential role of clinical care pathways in helping the clinical effectiveness process by trying them out in two directorates.
- Working with Pharmacy, the Drugs Committee, Microbiology and other service departments (e.g. X-ray) which are in a position to influence behaviour and thus improve clinical effectiveness.
- Seeking the use of clinical performance indicators in at least two directorates which will be:
  - a. directorate specific
  - b. locally trusted
  - c. generated automatically by working with Clinical Information Services.

- Working with the Medical Director to develop a sound system of resource focus whereby services of less proved effectiveness or less added value (most cost ineffective) are stopped or reduced.
- Influencing the development of Trust clinical information systems and using those to give information on practice.
- Ensuring that directorate programmes for clinical effectiveness (including education, information usage and audit) are part of the Trust business plan.

Monitor

> The NHS must monitor these changes locally in order to demonstrate real improvements in the quality, effectiveness and cost-effectiveness of health care[3].

It is essential for clinicians and managers to work with their colleagues in Corporate Information Services to dovetail each other's skills and ensure that the quality of data collection and interpretation is both accurate and appropriate for the purpose. This is occurring by:

- Working with the Risk Management Group to set up a monitoring system for clinical incident reporting.
- Ensuring high impact directorate audit programmes are part of the Trust business plan.
- Setting up and influencing the organisation of the Trust-wide clinical audit programme which is orientated towards:

  a. monitoring patient-related outcomes
  b. Trust-wide issues affecting clinical performance
  c. addressing issues of inappropriate resources use.

  This will entail the establishment of a rolling programme of five Trust-wide audits which will be a first priority on the use of the clinical effectiveness team resource.

- Maintenance of a record of the Trust's performance against the National Clinical Indicators.
- Setting up of a system to examine the impact of the Clinical Effectiveness Strategy.

A collaborative approach to clinical audit strategy for community health care

Sue Trinder, Oxfordshire Multidisciplinary Clinical Audit Advisory Group (MAAG)

For me the establishment of the Primary Care Quality Forum (PCQF) in 1996 made perfect sense. Service development, education and clinical audit were all well established in primary care, but seemed to function independently, with little indication of approach and effort. Several disparate groups were involved. It was becoming increasingly clear that our roles were overlapping and that there was an opportunity for us to coordinate our work and benefit from each other's skills and strengths. The PCQF was formed to be the main multidisciplinary coordinating forum for all those working towards improving quality in primary care. It brings together the MAAG, Professional Development Group (PDG) and others, as shown in Figure 8.5. We have agreed a mission statement ('To improve the quality of primary health care services by fostering the development, dissemination and implementation of good practice in Oxfordshire primary health care teams'. All members of the PCQF participate in setting priorities, so that these balance everyone's interests.

Our current MAAG activities reflect the success of this union. For example, recently we ran a series of clinical effectiveness workshops on finding, critically appraising and implementing evidence in the management of one pre-chosen condition in primary care. The running of the workshops involved the MAAG, GP tutors, PDG, Public Health Specialist and the Librarian from the Institute of Health Sciences. There are various other examples of successful joint working, such as the production of a pack to assist practices in the secondary prevention of coronary heart disease.

The staff of the MAAG have continued to function as an executive group for promoting and developing primary care clinical audit within this broader setting of quality development. The PCQF has certainly changed my role as an audit facilitator for the MAAG. I now have a much wider remit and many more working links with specialists from other fields.

I believe that clinical audit is gaining its rightful place in primary care as an integral part of the development of Oxfordshire's Primary Health Care Teams (PHCTs) and is no longer seen as 'something else to do' and separate from practice development.

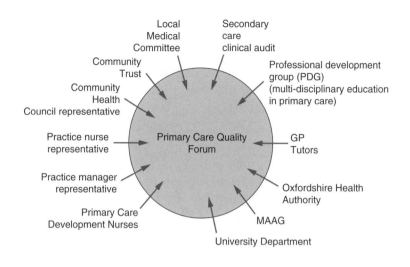

Figure 8.5 **The Primary Care Quality Forum (PCQF).**

Looking at the systems and structures within your own organisation draw a diagram of how these fit together at strategic, organisational and clinical levels to sustain the development of clinical audit.

Reviewing the clinical audit programme

As described in Chapter 5, the NHS Executive funded the development of a Clinical Audit Assessment Framework[4], which provides a description of good practice for clinical audit programmes and can be used to review and assess clinical audit activities across an organisation. The framework for assessing and improving a clinical audit programme parallels that for clinical audit projects. It is recommended that data are collected around three questions:

- How are topics for audit identified and selected?
- What impact has the audit programme had on the organisation and the health care it provides?
- What does the audit programme cost?

The programme assessment framework offers seven areas for further investigation:

- management and direction
- planning
- support and resources
- coverage and participation
- training and skills development
- monitoring and reporting
- evaluation.

This structured review forms the basis for planning changes to the clinical audit programme with a view to making it more effective in future. The detailed proforma can be found in Appendix 5.

Clinical audit: a commissioning perspective

About commissioning

Since the NHS reforms of the 1990s (NHS and Community Care Act 1990) the purchasing of health care has been separated from provision with purchasing being undertaken by Health Authorities, GP fundholders and total purchasing pilots. From 1991 to 1998 the NHS operated as an 'internal market'.

During the 1990s the wider definition of commissioning has replaced purchasing. Commissioning is a process whereby:

- assessment is made of the health needs of the population
- health priorities are determined
- health aims and strategies are developed
- service planning with health service providers and other organisations (such as local authority departments) is undertaken
- agreements and contracts are placed and monitored
- evaluation of the health impact of the population is assessed[6].

Commissioners are responsible for improving the health of their population by activities including the purchasing of high quality, cost effective health services for that population.

Measuring quality

A major criticism of the internal market was that cost effectiveness was the dominant determinant with less priority given to quality. Quality in health care proved difficult to measure and thus the focus was often on activity that could be more easily . counted. Over the course of the 1990s systems were devised which allowed more meaningful measures of quality. Health Commissioners included quality standards for both clinical and non-clinical quality in contracts. Amongst these a key tool for measurement of clinical quality is clinical audit.

As outlined in Chapter 1, recent government policy changes have raised the profile of quality in health care, introducing a statutory responsibility for quality in the form of clinical governance[7,8].

Commissioners and clinical audit

Aims Health service commissioners aim to commission services that are clinically effective and cost efficient and are appropriate and acceptable to their local population. Recently there has been increasing development of the clinical effectiveness/ evidence-based health care agenda and commissioners have taken this forward in part by linking this to clinical audit programmes.

Commissioners thus aim to use the clinical audit programme to improve quality. Specific purposes include monitoring local service quality and outcomes against evidence-based standards, benchmarking local services against other comparable populations nationally, agreeing and monitoring priorities for quality improvement, determining local 'lifelong learning needs' and influencing future commissioning decisions.

Resources Health Authority commissioners have been responsible for agreeing with local providers the use of initially 'ring fenced' and latterly locally agreed resources for clinical audit. In general, an arrangement has been agreed whereby 40% of resources are allocated to commissioner priority audit, 40% to Trust priority audit, 10% to primary/secondary care interface audits and 10% for other projects. Funding for clinical audit thus encompasses medical, nursing and professional clinical services projects.

In primary care audit activity is funded and coordinated via Medical Audit Advisory Groups (MAAGS) who support practitioners in primary care, including Practice Nurses, to conduct clinical audit.

Additionally, Trusts are required or opt to participate in national and/or regional audit and commissioners encourage such activity and have an interest in the results.

A partnership programme for effectiveness and audit

VIV Bennett, Quality Manager, Birmingham Health Authority

In Birmingham this agenda is being taken forward by the Birmingham Effectiveness Group. Established by the Health Authority this group comprises the Medical Director from each Trust, the MAAG and General Practice and professional advisors for nursing and pharmacy. It promotes clinical effectiveness and evidence-based commissioning and works through subgroups for priority topics that engage a range of health care professionals.

Local priority topics are determined and all Trusts providing the services involved participate in the programme. Audit methodologies are agreed and results reported at least annually.

Example

For the years 1996–8 the priority topics were:

■ management of back pain
■ post operative pain control following day surgery
■ anti-coagulation for atrial fibrillation
■ early treatment for meningitis with penicillin
■ use of steroids in preterm labour
■ pressure sores
■ issues in schizophrenia management.

These topics involved engagement of key professionals from a number of disciplines across the 11 local Trusts and from primary care. For some, e.g. steroids in preterm labour, evidence-based guidelines and national targets are available. Audit was undertaken to establish performance against these to enable Trusts to identify where and how improvements should be made. For others, for example pressure sores, a local statement of good practice based on currently available evidence and 'expert opinion' was agreed; this will enable consistent monitoring of incidence to take place and suggest improved management. Meningitis is an area of high public concern nationally. The project requires each Trust to have in place a protocol for early treatment with penicillin and to audit compliance. The subject of pain management post-day surgery included patients' views on how well their pain was relieved and highlighted a number of areas where management can be improved.

Implementation

The challenge for this programme and indeed for clinical audit in general is to implement the findings and where necessary to change practice. Local ownership and links with continuing professional education must be established. The reinforcement that all health care professionals have a responsibility to audit practice is essential, as is the notion that all members of a team, including clinical and non clinical support, have a contribution to make to implementing recommendations arising from audit to improve services.

The future

Whilst the arrangements for commissioning will change with the development of local commissioning groups there remains a responsibility for those commissioning as well as those providing health services to ensure that systems for quality and audit are in place and are robust. The new NHS intends to move from annual contracts to longer term service agreements. Commissioners working within health improvement plans and national service frameworks will be required to develop standards-based approaches to these agreements. A robust clinical audit programme agreed between commissioners and providers will be an essential component ensuring that the local population has access to high quality health care services.

Find out about the negotiations with commissioners who hold the budgets for clinical audit in your organisation. How are priorities decided? What opportunity is there for staff input?

Summary

- The facilitator plays a role in establishing supportive organisational structures which enable the implementation of clinical audit.
- Depending on the scale and the focus of the programme, different levels of facilitation may be required to support the strategic, organisational and clinical issues of implementation.
- Strategic issues are primarily concerned with the strategy of the implementation process and involve the careful integration of several initiatives.
- Organisational issues focus on developing systems and structures to support the implementation process of the clinical audit programme.
- Clinical issues involve teams working together at a local level to make clinical audit happen in practice.
- Clinical audit programmes require regular review.
- Clinical audit programmes need to be planned in partnership with health service commissioners.

References

1 Adair J 1987 Effective teambuilding. Pan Books, London
2 Heron J 1989 The facilitator's handbook. Kogan Page, London
3 Department of Health / NHS Executive 1996 Promoting clinical effectiveness: a framework for action in and through the NHS. HMSO, London, p 7
4 Walshe K, Spurgeon P 1997 Clinical Audit Assessment Framework. HSMC Handbook series 24, University of Birmingham
5 Department of Health 1993 Clinical audit in the HCHC: allocation of funds 1993/4. EL 93(34), NHSME, Leeds
6 Overtveit J 1995 Purchasing for health. A multidisciplinary introduction to the theory and practice of health purchasing. Open University Press, Buckingham
7 Department of Health 1997 The new NHS. Modern. Dependable. HMSO, London
8 Department of Health 1998 A first class service: quality in the new NHS. HMSO, London

9

Towards effective health care

The final chapter examines the role of clinical audit in relation to the many other activities and systems which seek to promote effective health care. Integrating clinical audit within the wider organisation is a theme which recurs throughout this book as it is considered critical to its success. This chapter describes clinical audit in the context of:

- quality improvement
- clinical effectiveness
- research
- continuing professional education.

Clinical audit and quality improvement

> Do not rely on audit to achieve improvement. Rely instead, on an overall system for improvement within which audit has a limited, albeit necessary role[1].

You may be familiar with the term quality assurance, which implies that a certain level or standard of service can be guaranteed. Quality improvement is about constantly looking at ways of doing things better – developing the standards achieved as time goes on. It involves creative problem-solving or looking for bright ideas as to how the service provided can be developed.

As you will know from your own experience, if the entire organisation is not committed to a new development, things will not change. Experience suggests that clinical audit is most effective when it forms a part of a coherent strategy for quality[2].

You will have heard terms such as continuous quality, total quality, or quality improvement. These all convey a 'philosophy' of improvement which is entirely complementary to, if not essential for, the successful implementation of clinical audit, as described at the end of Chapter 1. An organisational commitment to quality emphasises the links between departments and the need for everybody to take responsibility for quality. Within health care settings, unless every person within every department takes quality seriously, it is not possible to deliver an excellent service to the patient. The relationship between the various approaches to quality improvement and other related activities needs to be carefully considered and clearly set out within a strategy for the organisation.

In its 1994 publication, 'The evolution of clinical audit', the Department of Health makes it clear that clinical audit is to be developed with explicit links to other related activities.

> Clinical audit is not an isolated activity. It should be developed from existing clinical quality initiatives. Both health professionals and general managers should seek ways to harness other quality improvement programmes including Continuous Quality Improvement (CQI), and Total Quality Management (TQM)[3].

Many of these ideas have come from experience of improving quality in industry. The transfer of these principles and ideas to the public sector has been discussed and these authors cite the American Federal Office of Management and Budget Circular which defines Total Quality Management as 'a total organisational approach for meeting customer needs and expectations that involves all managers and employees in using quantitative methods to improve continuously the organisation's processes, products and services'[4].

Many health care organisations are looking for external approval of their commitment to quality improvement. There are many models of approval in use and these range from systems whose focus is staff development and training, such as Investors in People, to adaptations of industrial quality systems, for example the ISO 9000 series. The International Standards Organisation (ISO) is the parent organisation of the British Standards Institute – you will remember the BSI kitemark. The ISO 9000 series gives organisations the opportunity to be 'kitemarked' by showing assessors that they have a comprehensive set of systems in place to assure the standard of the services they provide.

There is increasing interest in a framework provided by the European Foundation for Quality Management (EFQM). This has been developed in Europe from the Malcolm Baldridge Award Framework in the USA. The EFQM model for excellence claims to be a 'non-prescriptive framework based on nine criteria, which can be used to assess an organisation's progress towards excellence'[5].

Another externally applied quality system developed specifically for health care is the King's Fund Organisational Audit (now called Health Quality Service) (see details in Appendix 2). This is based on a framework of explicit standards concerned with the organisation and management of health care services. It is clear how it fits in with clinical audit as it requires a written clinical audit schedule linked to organisational priorities; a mechanism for staff and patients to make suggestions for audit topics; that audit takes place across disciplines; that records are kept of audit meetings; and that recommendations from audit are implemented. Other systems include the Hospital Accreditation Programme and Health Services Accreditation.

There remains a debate about how external accreditation systems fit with improvement-based approaches to quality and clinical audit. The reality within a complex organisation is that there is a need to assure standards of care whilst at the same time seeking to improve. It is important to be clear within an organisation about which systems are being used for which purpose. In addition, attention should be given to the way in which these systems are used. A system based on external assessment can be implemented in a way which retains the principles of quality improvement by involving staff as partners and ensuring that they take an active part in the whole process.

Develop a list of initiatives within your organisation which you consider should be included in a strategy for quality.

Find out about the quality strategy in your organisation:
—Does it include all the items on your list?
—How could it be improved?
Write a quality strategy for your department.

Summary

- Quality improvement is about constantly seeking to do better.
- Clinical audit cannot exist in isolation, it must form an integral part of an organisation's strategy for quality.
- Organisations may have a range of systems in place to assure and improve quality. These should all reflect a philosophy of staff involvement and ownership.

Clinical audit, guidelines and clinical effectiveness

As mentioned in the introduction, clinical audit is increasingly being recognised as a practical tool for implementing research findings in practice. Clinical effectiveness is defined as 'the application of the best available knowledge, derived from research, clinical expertise and patient preferences to achieve optimum processes and outcomes of care for patients'[6].

Clinical effectiveness encompasses research, the provision and critical appraisal of evidence including clinical guidelines, education and training, involving patients or patient organisations, risk management, national monitoring of health outcome indicators as well as clinical audit. All these initiatives come together in an attempt to ensure that decisions about the provision and delivery of health care are based on the very best of available evidence about clinical and cost effectiveness, alongside the monitoring of actual health outcomes[7], as shown in Figure 9.1.

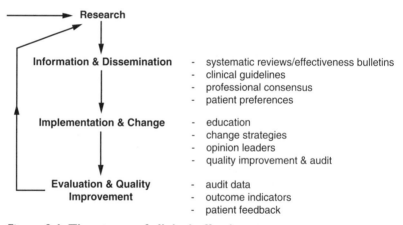

Figure 9.1 The stages of clinical effectiveness.

Therefore, as well as forming a part of an organisation's quality strategy, clinical audit can be seen as one part of a larger programme of clinical effectiveness. Clinical audit provides a means of clinical staff translating the information generated at a national level into meaningful standards which can then be implemented, informing the development of care to a group of patients or clients.

National clinical guidelines are particularly closely allied to clinical audit. They are defined as 'systematically developed statements to assist practitioner and patient decisions about appropriate health care for specific circumstances[8]. If the guidelines are based on good evidence they can inform the standards against which practice is measured.

Guidelines are developed by a number of agencies. Often one agency will take the lead and others will collaborate. Issues may be chosen for guideline development because they are an area of concern to professionals or patient groups and this is usually because there is a wide variation in practice across the UK. Some examples of agencies that have developed national clinical guidelines appear in Table 9.1.

Table 9.1 Approaches to solving clinical practice issues

Category of agency	Example agency	Guideline example
Medical Royal Colleges	Royal College of General Practitioners	Clinical Guidelines for the Management of Acute Low Back Pain
Other professional bodies	Chartered Society of Physiotherapy	Guideline for the early treatment of the hand after injury or surgery
Self-help and support groups	National Childbirth Trust	Guidelines for the management of treatment and testing of newborns with hypoglycaemia
Academic institutions	University of Newcastle upon Tyne	Guidelines for the use of ACE inhibitors in patients with heart failure (in progress)
Collaborative agencies	Scottish Intercollegiate Guidelines Network (SIGN)	Obesity in Scotland

However good national clinical guidelines may appear it is important to appraise them for yourselves. An appraisal instrument has been produced by a team led from St George's Hospital Medical School[9] to assist practitioners in this process. It provides criteria against which to consider issues such as the rigour of the guideline development, i.e. its coverage, reliability and reproducibility, and whether a multi-professional group has been involved in its development.

Guidelines are written in a variety of formats and often need adapting to form the basis of a clinical audit project. National clinical guidelines may be formulated in such a way that they naturally form objectives for the desired quality of service. Equally they may provide the level of detail which could provide criteria against which practice can be measured. As well as modifying the format of a national clinical guideline, the content may also need adapting to provide a standard which is specific to a particular clinical unit. However, care must be taken not to pick and choose recommendations to suit the local situation in a way that undermines the evidence on which the guidelines are based. Having customised the guidelines, their recommendations can then be implemented prior to moving onto the measurement phase of clinical audit. Box 9.1 summarises the issues to be considered when adapting nationally written guidelines for local use.

Box 9.1 Adapting nationally written guidelines for local use[11]

Preparation
- Find out who else is interested in improving a particular aspect of care and set up an audit/improvement team
- Decide the roles and responsibilities of team members
- Enlist management support for your project
- Find out if anyone you work with has specialist knowledge of the topic of interest
- Locate clinical guidelines: central databases, libraries, NHSE, professional organisations
- Make sure everyone understands the terms and concepts used in the national guidelines

Local interpretation
- Check that the recommendations made in the guideline are achievable in your workplace
- Check that the recommendations are achievable with the people you work with
- Check that each guideline is desirable for the clients and staff you work with
- Find out the views of clients and staff
- Agree what needs to be changed to make the guideline achievable
- Agree what needs to be changed to make it desirable

> **Box 9.1 Adapting nationally written guidelines for local use[10] (contd.)**
>
> ■ Establish which recommendations are mandatory and which are optional, based on the grading of the evidence presented
> ■ Look to see whether possible choices for adapting recommendations locally are given with rationales to assist your decision-making
> ■ Assemble all the information you need to make adaptations, e.g. research literature, local policies, etc.
> ■ Make adaptations to enable guidelines to be implemented locally

Guidelines can be a useful tool within the commissioning process. Commissioners may ask individual Trusts to devise clinical audit projects using national clinical guidelines as a basis[11]. Other publications which make research evidence available include Effective Health Care Bulletins, Effectiveness Matters, and systematic reviews of research evidence. Further details of providers of information can be found in Appendix 2. These may also provide useful evidence to develop standards and criteria against which to measure practice.

The relationship between national clinical guidelines and clinical audit works both ways. It has been suggested that audit results highlighting variation in practice have influenced the development of increasing numbers of guidelines[12]. The issues raised by audit help to inform the priorities for research, as illustrated in Figure 9.1, which may then be used as the basis for national clinical guidelines.

Increasingly, organisations are establishing research and development committees and programmes which in many areas have been combined or clearly linked with the clinical audit strategies and structures. Clinical effectiveness provides an opportunity to bring together research, development, education, guidelines and clinical audit. As discussed in the previous section it is important to remember that the implementation of clinical effectiveness is enhanced by linking it into an organisational strategy for quality improvement[13] including clinical governance.

Within the literature on evidence-based care and clinical effectiveness terms are from time to time used slightly differently.

Words such as protocol, guideline, standard may be used in very similar ways. In order to minimise confusion it is important to take note of the context in which they are being used, but most importantly to assess the quality of the evidence on which they are based and then to adapt them into whatever format is most familiar or useful. Research, however, has a distinct role and should not be confused with clinical audit. This is the subject of the next section.

Find out about the clinical effectiveness programme in your organisation.
What national clinical guidelines exist within your field of care?
—On what evidence are they based?

Summary

- Clinical audit needs to be integrated within a programme of clinical effectiveness.
- Clinical audit should be based upon the best available evidence.
- Where national clinical guidelines exist they should be used as a basis for clinical audit.

Clinical audit and research

Clinical audit and research have complementary roles to play in ensuring clinical effectiveness. There is, however, some confusion over whether research and audit are one and the same activity. Many authors have tried to make clear distinctions. Most commonly the difference is described in terms of research determining the right thing to do and that the role of audit is to determine whether the right thing is actually done[14]. The purpose of research has been described as 'to add to a general body of scientific knowledge which has universal application', and the purpose of clinical audit as 'to enable practitioners to monitor and improve practice in specific situations'[15].

There has been some debate as to whether audit needs to be carried out with the same rigour as research. One view is that 'unless audit is seen by the health professions as a rigorous discipline that itself sets high standards in the pursuit of worthwhile benefits for patients and professionals it will surely fail to deliver improvements in quality'[16]. This needs to be balanced with the importance of audit as an activity owned by practitioners at local level to improve the quality of care in their particular settings.

You may have encountered action research which is becoming increasingly popular in health care. It is defined as a 'type of self reflective enquiry undertaken by participants in social situations in order to improve the rationality and justice of their own practices, their understandings of these practices and the situations in which these practices are carried out'[17]. This field of research shows the most similarities to clinical audit. It has been suggested that although action research and clinical audit both aim to improve the quality of care and follow a cyclical process, their emphasis is different. 'Action researchers emphasise professional, personal and group development through educative and democratic processes and action research is frequently used to generate theories'[18]. Clinical audit in contrast is seen to be focused on customer requirements and the findings from clinical audit are not used to generate theory.

Four links between clinical audit and research have been identified[19]. Firstly, research informing the clinical audit process by providing the evidence for standards and criteria against which practice is measured. Secondly, clinical audit informing research where the results of audit provoke the sorts of discussion that lead to the formulation of new research questions. Thirdly, the application of research methods in clinical audit. The confusion between the two activities stems from their similar appearance because of the contribution of research methods to clinical audit[20]. Those familiar with the principles of research will recognise the same process in designing an audit project – literature review, sampling, design of data collection tools, piloting data collection tools, consideration of validity and reliability, data analysis and report writing.

The fourth link is using research to evaluate the effectiveness of audit so that the process of audit itself is examined and evaluated on a national level. Between 1989 and 1995, the NHS Executive provided £279 million for the introduction and development of medical and clinical audit in the NHS[21] in England. Various reports and evaluations of the programme have been commissioned to evaluate the effect clinical audit has had on clinical practice and patient care[12,22–26].

There has been increasing emphasis in recent years on linking research and development to education. The same is true of clinical audit and this is the subject of the next section.

Identify three differences between research and audit.
Design a diagram to show how research, guidelines and audit fit into your clinical effectiveness strategy locally.

Summary

- Research and clinical audit are distinct activities with complementary roles to play in clinical effectiveness.
- Although different, action research has particular similarities to clinical audit.
- Research methods can be applied to audit.

Clinical audit, education and professional development

Participation in audit is a particularly useful way to identify learning needs: whether for the person, the clinical team or the organisation[3].

When audit was first introduced it was perceived by the medical profession as an educational tool. 'Effective audit and effective education contribute to the same process. At a personal level, this is the process of facilitating individual critical appraisal as a part of professional development: adult learning requires educational needs assessment, audit provides the clinical standards assessment on which to improve the quality of care[27].' In a recent review of the use of the Dynamic Standard Setting System[2] it was clear that the development of practice and the development of practitioners were inextricably linked.

It has been suggested that education and training need to be addressed at three stages: before, during and as a result of the audit[28]. Audit can have significant educational value depending on the composition of the groups, choice of audit topics, and the skills with which meetings are facilitated and conducted. Clinical audit provides a mechanism that encourages health care professionals to reflect upon their work in order to develop their practice, knowledge and attitudes[29,30].

For nurses this process of reflection on practice can be structured as a part of the process of re-registration with the UKCC. This is known as PREP (post registration education and practice) and it enables nurses to demonstrate how their learning influences the development of clinical practice. Involvement in clinical audit is an appropriate means of fulfilling these requirements.

Clinical audit can enhance the continuing professional development of all clinical staff. Continuing professional development is defined as the 'maintenance and enhancement of knowledge, expertise and competence of professionals throughout their career according to a plan formulated with regard to the needs of the professional, the employer, the profession and society'[31]. Continuing professional development can be contrasted with traditional continuing education as it encompasses a broader view of the skills needed in health care practice and would include the following[32]:

- Acquisition/application of new knowledge
- Better application of existing knowledge
- Enhanced management of health care
  working as a team
  working within the organisation
- Enhanced communication
  with patients
  within the clinical team
  between clinical teams
  with managers
- Improved teaching skills
- Attention to social, cultural, ethical and psychological aspects of care
- Use of information technology
- Maturation of the individual, the team and the organisation.

This concept of learning extending to the team and the organisation is echoed throughout the literature. The term 'learning organisation'[33] describes the necessary dimensions for building organisations which can learn. This willingness throughout an organisation to learn and develop is sometimes referred to as organisational culture. In an evaluation of medical audit in provider units in England[12] 'audit was reported to have contributed to changing the culture of health care providers, developing a greater sense of clinical accountability, openness, inter-professional understanding and sensitivity to patients' needs'.

It has also been suggested that 'audit is emerging as a strategically invaluable space for significant learning. It shows potential for harnessing the creativity required to find ways of jointly managing competing accountabilities so as to produce clinically effective services'[34].

At a practical level, it appears that learning occurs throughout the audit cycle; when researching the evidence on which to base standards, in the implementation phase, in the development of measuring tools, the collection of data, action planning and throughout the process as the multi-professional group learns to work more effectively together and collaborate within the wider organisation.

The following example shows how research, clinical audit and education have been integrated to enhance patient care.

Using research, audit and education to minimise the risk of drug administration errors

Jill Gladstone, Clinical Audit Coordinator, Royal Devon and Exeter Healthcare NHS Trust

Drug administration constitutes one of the highest risk areas of nursing care and a drug error is likely to be the adverse clinical event most feared by practising nurses. In its entirety, drug administration consists of a complex chain of events, involving different members of staff and several professional groups. Drug errors may arise as a result of a fault at any part of this chain. From a risk management point of view, a drug error is likely to be legally indefensible.

The Royal Devon and Exeter Healthcare NHS Trust has used a programme combining research, audit and education to:

- ensure safe and accurate drug administration to patients
- improve clinical practice in the multi-professional team
- provide evidence to support the planning and implementation of educational input and managerial changes.

Methods

Both clinical audit projects and research projects employed a range of qualitative and quantitative techniques.

- Clinical audit projects demonstrated poor standards of prescription writing, poor use of infusion device resources, inadequate drug policies, lack of compliance by a rapidly changing population of nurses and doctors.
- Research identified confusion regarding defining and reporting drug errors, fear of disciplinary action and lack of updating in drug administration skills.

Outcomes

- Improved standard of prescription writing and heightened awareness of its importance
- Centralisation of infusion devices into a pump bank and more effective management of these resources
- Implementation of new drug administration policies
- Review of pre and postregistration education programmes relating to drug administration
- Introduction of a Trust-wide policy for managing and supporting nurses involved in drug incidents.

How could involvement in clinical audit help you fulfil your personal learning objectives?
What learning needs do you perceive for your team or organisation?

Summary

- Clinical audit enhances the professional development of those involved.
- Clinical audit provides opportunities for learning in teams.
- Clinical audit encourages a process of reflection upon practice.

Moving forward

A range of benefits of involvement in clinical audit can be identified, including increased reflection on the quality of clinical care delivered, developments in team-building and collaboration, the implementation of changes in clinical practice, and improvements in patient experiences and patient outcomes of care.

As organisations are able to integrate clinical audit, clinical governance, clinical effectiveness, research and development into organisational quality strategies it is hoped that these activities will be more closely integrated into the everyday working practices of clinical teams, minimising the extra time involved. Just as organisations have a responsibility to establish strategies with supporting systems and structures to enable clinical audit, so clinical staff have a responsibility to commit themselves to improving clinical care.

You have now completed the clinical audit handbook. You may now wish to discuss your thoughts and ideas with your colleagues as you seek to influence the further development of clinical audit locally. It is hoped that you now feel confident to work systematically through a clinical audit project whilst ensuring that your project is clearly linked into other related initiatives within your organisation. We wish you every success!

References

1. Berwick DM 1992 Heal thyself or heal thy system: can doctors help to improve medical care? Quality in Healthcare 11(suppl): 2–8
2. Morrell C, Harvey G, Kitson AL 1995 The reality of practitioner based quality improvement, report no. 14. National Institute for Nursing, Oxford
3. Department of Health 1994 The evolution of clinical audit. DoH, London, p10, p17
4. Morgan C, Murgatroyd S 1994 Total quality management in the public sector. Open University Press, Buckingham
5. The RCN Clinical Effectiveness Initiative: a strategic framework. RCN, London
6. RCN 1996 clinical effectiveness strategy. Clinical effectiveness steering group
7. NHSE 1996 Promoting clinical effectiveness. DoH, London
8. Institute for Medicine 1992 Guidelines for clinical practice: from development to use. National Academic Press, Washington, DC
9. Cluzeau F, Littlejohns P, Grimshaw J, Feder G 1997 Appraisal instrument for clinical guidelines, HCEU. St George's Hospital Medical School, London
10. Duff LA, Kitson AL, Watson R, Edgson R, Bakewell J 1993 Standards of Nutrition and the Older Adult: A report on the development of national standards for the nutritional care of older adults in continuing care. Royal College of Nursing, DQI Programme, Oxford
11. Humphris D, Littlejohns P 1996 The development of multi-professional audit and clinical guidelines: their contribution to quality assurance and the effectiveness of the NHS. Journal of Interprofessional Care (9)3: 207–225
12. Buttery Y, Walshe K, Coles J, Bennett J 1994 The Development of Audit. CASPE Research, London

13. Humphris D, Littlejohns P 1996 Implementing clinical guidelines: preparation and opportunism. Journal of Clinical Effectiveness (1)1: 5–7
14. Smith R 1992 Audit and research. BMJ 305: 905–906
15. Closs SJ, Cheater FM 1996 Audit or research – what is the difference? Journal of Clinical Nursing 5: 249–256
16. Russell IT, Wilson BJ 1992 Audit the third clinical science? Quality in Health Care 1(1): 51–55
17. Carr W, Kemmis S 1986 Becoming critical. Falmer, London
18. Waterman H 1996 A comparison between quality assurance and action research. Nurse Researcher 3(3): 58–68
19. Harvey G 1996 Relating quality assessment and audit to the research process in nursing. Nurse Researcher 3(3): 35–46
20. Balogh R 1996 Exploring the links between audit and the research process. Nurse Researcher 3(3): 5–16
21. National Audit Office 1995 Clinical audit in England. HMSO, London
22. Walshe K, Coles J 1993 A review of initiatives. CASPE Research, London
23. Willmott M, Foster J 1995 A review of audit activity in the nursing and therapy professions. CASPE Research, London
24. Stern M, Brennan S 1993 Medical audit in the hospital and community health service. Department of Health, London
25. von Degenberg K 1994 Clinical audit in the nursing and therapy professions. Department of Health, London
26. Clinical Outcomes Group 1994 Clinical audit in primary health care. Department of Health, London
27. Houghton G 1996 Linking clinical audit and continuing medical education. Audit Trends 4(1): 1–2
28. Vimpany M, Nixon K 1995 Reflections on education and audit. Audit Trends 3(4): 137–139
29. Schon D 1991 The reflective practitioner: how professionals think in action. Avebury, Aldershot
30. Argyris C 1993 Teaching smart people how to learn. In: Howard R (ed) The learning imperative: managing people for continuous innovation. Harvard Business School Press, Boston
31. Madden C, Mitchell V 1993 Professions, standards and competence – a survey of continuing education for the professions. Bristol, University of Bristol, Department for Continuing Education
32. Batstone G, Edwards M 1994 Clinical audit – how do we proceed? Southampton Medical Journal Jan 1994, 13–19
33. Senge P 1990 The fifth discipline – the art and practice of the learning organisation. Century Press, London
34. Weil SW 1994 Enhancing clinical effectiveness: stimulating and sustaining organisational capacity for significant learning. Discussion paper for NHS Executive Clinical Outcomes Group 2.12.94

Glossary

Clinical audit   a clinically led initiative which seeks to improve the quality and outcome of patient care. This is achieved through the multi-professional team together examining and modifying their practices according to standards of what could be achieved, based on the best available evidence. (Adapted from Mann)[1].

Clinician   any health care professional.

Clinical effectiveness   'the application of the best available knowledge, derived from research, clinical expertise and patient preferences to achieve optimum processes and outcomes of care for patients'[2].

Clinical guidelines   'systematically developed statements to assist practitioner and patient decisions about appropriate health care for specific circumstances'[3].

Criterion based audit   involves identifying specific measurable criteria for the achievement of good practice which can be compared with what actually happens.

Criterion   an item necessary to and indicative of the achievement of an objective.

Objective   a broad statement of good practice based on the best possible evidence.

Protocol   offers explicit step-by-step guidance for clinical staff for a specific aspect of clinical care. It is developed locally, often adapted from a nationally prepared clinical guideline, and should always be based on the best available evidence. Protocols are often referred to in the criteria of a standard. In some areas a protocol may be called a local guideline.

Standard   'outlines an objective with guidance for its achievement given in the form of criteria sets which specify required resources, activities and predicted outcomes'[4]. This is the overarching term used to describe what is being aimed for.

References

1. Mann T 1996 Clinical audit in the NHS. NHSE, Leeds
2. RCN 1996 The RCN Clinical Effectiveness Initiative: a strategic framework. RCN, London
3. Institute for Medicine 1992 Guidelines for clinical practice: from development to use. National Academic Press, Washington, DC
4. Royal College of Nursing 1990 Quality patient care – the Dynamic Standard Setting System. Scutari, Harrow

Appendix I

Code of conduct for clinical audit

All researchers employed by, or attached to, the RCN Institute abide by a written code of conduct which commits them to protect the interests of all actual and potential data providers. The following is an adaptation of that code of conduct for clinical audit groups and *applies when clinical audit involves directly interviewing or giving questionnaires to potential data providers.*

The code is based on five main principles:

1. *Clarifying/justifying the purpose of clinical audit.* Before each potential data provider is asked to provide the Clinical Audit Group with information, he or she is told why the clinical audit project is being undertaken, who has commissioned it, the possible uses of the information and the availability of the final document.

2. *Informed consent.* Following the more general explanation of the purpose of the audit project, the auditor gives an explanation of the nature of the data collection. The auditor explains to the data provider how the data are to be used.

3. *Ensuring anonymity.* Before each potential data provider is asked to impart information, he or she is given a guarantee that no information will be passed on to any third party other than in such a form that it cannot be attributed to the data provider.

4. *Safeguarding confidentiality.* Each data provider is given a guarantee by the Clinical Audit Group that no information provided will be used other than for the purpose of the clinical audit project and its dissemination.

5. *Respecting the privacy of the data providers.* Even when a data provider has accepted the guarantees of informed consent, anonymity and confidentiality, the Clinical Audit Group are obliged to ensure that any data collection is carried out following negotiation and full discussion with the

subject. Each encounter should be executed in such a way as to minimise any sense of intrusion of the auditor into the life of the data provider. The data provider should be reminded that at any time he or she may opt out of the encounter.

Each principle demands a number of practical procedures in order to ensure that the clinical audit project is carried out in an acceptable way.

Clarifying/justifying the purpose of the clinical audit project

The Clinical Audit Group must ensure:

- production of clear explanation of the project written in non-technical terms
- where appropriate, explanation of who has funded the project and what will be done with the information.

Informed consent

The Clinical Audit Group member:

- identifies him/herself to the data provider and shows appropriate form of identification
- explains general purpose of the project (see above) and specific purpose of encounter with potential data provider
- discusses and guarantees confidentiality and anonymity
- discusses ownership of data until the time of its agreed validation
- ensures that the data provider is aware that he or she can terminate the involvement with the project at any time
- discusses methods of data collection and practical implications of their use.

Ensuring anonymity

The Clinical Audit Group are responsible for the data collection storage systems that take account of the following factors:

- separation of names of data providers/wards/hospitals and other care settings from information provided

- development of a secure coding system known only by relevant personnel regarding data provider codes (see Box A1.1)
- ensuring that access to data is limited to authorised people only – tape transcribers, data collectors, data punchers (see Box A1.2)
- ensuring safe transfer of data from one area to another, particularly where data are moved from one institution to another, retaining tapes in a secure area when being transferred between transcribers and members of the Clinical Audit Group.

Safeguarding confidentiality

The Clinical Audit Group:

- are aware of the relevant passages in the Data Protection Act (1984)
- do not publish or pass to any third party any information which can be attributed to an individual
- know what to do with 'difficult' information received from the subject in confidence
- have worked through difficult issues such as ownership of information, e.g. does the data provider have a right to ask for confidential information to be destroyed?

Respecting welfare of data providers

The Clinical Audit Group:

- agree/negotiate times of meetings, place of meetings
- are sensitive to pressures of work and are willing to withdraw if situations are difficult
- do not intrude unreasonably into the daily work of data providers.

Each member of the Clinical Audit Group has a personal responsibility to ensure that these five requirements are met in the securing and handling of their data.

Box A1.1 Ensuring anonymity

Documents containing data collected from the data provider should be identified only by a number; however, a front cover sheet showing the name and address of a potential data provider involved in a project may be attached to a schedule before it is used. This sheet should be removed at the earliest opportunity. The master index linking the names and addresses of data providers to code numbers should be kept locked. If data documents or tapes have to be sent to a third party, for punching or transcribing, any cover sheets or other information that could link the document/tape to an individual must be removed or erased. Questionnaire returns, transcripts and all other documents, tapes and disks containing data from providers should be kept locked whenever possible. Keys should be available only to the relevant personnel. Data documents may be destroyed in accordance with the Data Protection Act.

In the case of a large project, where it is necessary to employ data collectors outside the Clinical Audit Group, and to temporarily store documents in a place other than the clinical audit office, it is the responsibility of the Clinical Audit Group to ensure that employees are aware of the confidential nature of the documents. Cover sheets with the names and addresses of data providers should be removed as soon as possible. Any documents linking individuals to data should be kept, where possible, in the Clinical Audit Office. If this is not possible, then they should be stored by the local data collector in a secure place. Data documents should be collected regularly to minimise the time they are outside the Clinical Audit Office.

Box A1.2 Anonymity of transcripts

I. Transcripts and cassette tapes containing interview data should be stored in a locked file.

II. The data provider codes should be locked in a separate data provider code file. Individual Clinical Audit Group members should be responsible for their own files and be the only people with access to the file.

III. Clinical Audit Group members are responsible for ensuring that secretaries transcribing tapes are aware of, and respect, the content of the ethical code.

IV. Transcribers of tapes working outside the Clinical Audit Office should sign a 'confidentiality of information' form when accepting tapes for transcription.

V. All transcripts should be transported to and from the Clinical Audit Office in boxes or envelopes marked CONFIDENTIAL.

Appendix 2

Sources of information

National guidelines

UK Clinical Audit Association
Room 9, Cleethorpes Centre
Jackson Place
Wilton Road
Humberston
South Humberside DN36 4AS
Tel: 01472 210 628
Has a database of published clinical guidelines for clinical care

Scottish Intercollegiate Network (SIGN)
Administration Support Group
Royal College of Physicians
9 Queen Street
Edinburgh EH2 1JQ
Tel: 0131 225 7324
web: http://pc47.cee.hw.ac.uk/sign/home.htm
Produces or supports the development of a variety of medically
related guidelines – list available on request

Academic centres of research and development – various speciality-related guidelines – for addresses and contacts see back
of recent publication: NHSE (1996) *Clinical Guidelines: using
guidelines to improve patient care within the NHS*, London,
NHSE; and NHSE (1997) *Clinical Effectiveness Resource Pack*,
London, NHSE

National speciality research bodies and groups – various
speciality-related guidelines. Consult librarian for various
directories containing appropriate names and addresses

Medical Royal Colleges – various speciality-related guidelines
largely produced by college research units.

Other professional bodies – various speciality-related guidelines. For addresses and contacts see back of publication: NHSE (1996) *Clinical Guidelines: using guidelines to improve patient care within the NHS*, London, NHSE. Alternatively contact the relevant professional body directly

Royal College of Nursing Dynamic Quality Improvement Programme
20 Cavendish Square
London W1M 0AB
Tel: 0171 409 3333
Involved in the production of clinical guidelines in various areas.

AHCPR
Agency for Health Care Policy and Research
PO Box 8547
Silver Spring
MD 20907
Tel: 001 800 358 9258, web: http://www.ahcpr.gov/
Produces a range of clinical guidelines – details of those published as of 1995 are available from the Nursing and Midwifery Audit Information Service (see page 176)

Try searching journals and databases such as MEDLINE/ Cinahl at your local hospital library or at national health libraries such as RCN library, King's Fund Library, but be aware of the rigour with which the guidelines have been produced, and do not assume that anything with guideline in the title is automatically of high quality.

Systematic reviews

NHSE Health Technology Assessments
Full list can be found in
NHSE (June 1996). *Report of the NHS Health Technology Assessment Programme 1996.*
Up-to-date information can be found from:
The National Co-ordinating Centre for Health Technology Assessment
Mailpoint 728, Boldrewood,
University of Southampton

Southampton SO16 7PX
Tel: 01703–595586
Email:hta@soton.ac.uk, web: http//www.soton.ac.uk/~hta

UK Cochrane Centre
The Cochrane Collaboration is an international network of individuals who help prepare, maintain and disseminate systematic reviews. They feed into the Cochrane Centre's regularly updated electronic journal, the Database of Systematic Reviews.
The UK Cochrane Centre
NHS R&D Programme,
Summertown Pavilion
Middle Way
Oxford OX2 7LG.
Tel: 01865 516300
Email: general@cochrane.co.uk,
web: http://hiru.mcmaster.ca/cochrane/default.html

NHS Centre for Reviews and Dissemination
Aims to carry out and commission reviews about the effectiveness of health care, maintain and update an international register of systematic reviews, produce guidelines and training material for those wishing to undertake systematic reviews, disseminate research-based information in a targeted way to decision-makers and consumers, and undertake research into effective dissemination. The NHS Centre for Reviews and Dissemination (CRD) is funded by the NHS Executive and the Health Departments of Scotland, Wales and Northern Ireland. The Centre compiles the Database of Abstracts of Reviews of Effectiveness (DARE). Also contact CRD for Effective Health Care Bulletins, Effectiveness Matters, National Research Register.
Information Services
The NHS Centre for Reviews and Dissemination
University of York
Heslington
York YO1 5DD
Tel: 01904 433707
web: http://www.york.ac.uk/inst/crd/welcome-htm

Centre for Evidence-Based Nursing
To facilitate the drive for evidence-based care the University of York has established a Centre for Evidence-Based Nursing as part of the national network of Centres for Evidence-Based Clinical Practice (which includes the Centre for Evidence-Based Medicine at Oxford and the Centre for Evidence-Based Child Health in London). Each Centre contributes a specific perspective. The Centre for Evidence-Based Nursing is working as part of this network, collaborating in the promotion of evidence-based health care.

The Centre for Evidence-Based Nursing works with nurses in practice, other researchers, nurse educators and managers to identify evidence-based practice through primary research and systematic reviews and promotes the uptake of evidence into practice through education and implementation activities in areas of nursing where good evidence is available. The Centre is also researching factors which promote or impede the implementation of evidence-based practice.
web: http://www.york.ac.uk/depts/hstd/centres/evidence/ev-intro.htm

Centre for Evidence-Based Medicine
Nuffield Department of Clinical Medicine
Level 5
The Oxford Radcliffe NHS Trust
Headley Way
Oxford OX3 9DU
Tel: 01865 222941

Centre for Evidence-Based Child Health
Department of Epidemiology
Institute of Child Health
30 Guildford Street
London W1CN 1EH
Tel: 0171 242 9783 x 2606
Email: cebch@irh.ud.ac.uk

CASP (Critical Appraisal Skills Programme)
Oxford Institute of Health Sciences
PO Box 777
Oxford OX3 7LF

Tel: 01865 226968
Fax: 01865 226959
Email: casp@cix.compulink.co.uk
web: http://www.ihs.ox.ac.uk/casp

Information on clinical audit

Nursing and Midwifery Audit Information Service
20 Cavendish Square
London W1M 0AB
Tel: 0171 647 3831
web: http//www.man.ac.uk/rcn/ukwide/nmais.htm
Database contains references to some nursing related and other guidelines

National Centre for Clinical Audit (NCCA)
The NCCA aims to provide enquirers with references from a catalogue of information available through a wide range of organisations and a large specialised database of audit references.
National Centre for Clinical Audit
Tavistock House
Tavistock Square
London WC1H 9JP
Tel: 0171 383 6451
Email: ncca@ncca.org.uk, web: http://www.ncca.org.uk

Clinical Effectiveness Support Unit Wales
Roseway
Llandough Hospital and Community NHS Trust
Penarth CF64 2XX
Tel 01222 716839
Fax 01222 716242
Email sesu@dial.pipex.com

At the time of going to press it is proposed that the National Centre for Clinical Excellence may assume many of the functions of the three resource centres listed above. The professional bodies and clinical effectiveness departments at NHS regions and boards will have up-to-date information.

Scottish Clinical Audit Resource Centre
The Scottish Clinical Audit Resource Centre was established in September 1994 with funding from the Clinical Resource and Audit Group. The remit of the Centre is to provide education, information and support to people taking part in audit throughout Scotland. The centre also carries out research into audit in Scotland.
Scottish Clinical Audit Resource Centre
Glasgow University
1 Horselethill Rd
Glasgow G12 9LX
Tel: 0141 330 6190
Fax: 0141 330 6192
E-mail: SCARC@pgm.gla.ac.uk

Eli Lilly National Clinical Audit Centre
The Lilly Audit Centre was created to be a national resource to health authorities, audit groups and others in the field of clinical audit. It is an integral part of the Department of General Practice and Primary Health Care at the University of Leicester and its principal remit is research and development of effective methods of clinical audit, particularly in the setting of primary health care and at the interface between primary and secondary care.

Eli Lilly National Clinical Audit Centre
Department of General Practice and Primary Health Care
University of Leicester
Leicester General Hospital
Gwendolen Road
Leicester LE5 4PW
Tel: 0116 258 4873
Fax: 0116 258 4982
Email: gpaudit@le.ac.uk, web: http://www.leicester.ac.uk/gpaudit/

Information on accreditation

The Health Quality Service
in association with The King's Fund
11-13 Cavendish Square
London W1M 0AN
Tel: 0171 307 2400
Fax: 0171 307 2804
Email:hqs@kehf.org.uk
web: www.kingsfund.org.uk

European Foundation for Quality Management
Brussells Representative Office
Avenue du Pleiades 15
1200 Brussells
Belgium
Tel: +32 2 775 3511
Fax: +32 2 775 3535
Email: info@efqm.org
web: http://www.efqm.org

For information on ISO 9000
British Standards Institute
389 Chiswick High Road
London W4 4AL
Tel: 0181 996 9000
web: www.bsi.org.uk

Internet sites

OMNI claims to be the UK's independent gateway to high quality biomedical Internet resources at web: http://omni.ac.uk/

Netting the Evidence with the University of Sheffield, Introduction to Evidence-Based Practice on the Internet, http://www.shef.ac.uk/uni/academic/R-Z/scharr/ir/netting.html

Appendix 3

Forms for clinical audit

This section contains:

- alternative layouts for standards
- a series of proformas for clinical audit
- a completed set of proformas.

Alternative layouts for standards

Example 1

STANDARD FORM*	
STANDARD REF:	IMPLEMENT BY:
TOPIC: Safety	AUDIT BY:
SUB-TOPIC: Administration of Medicines	SIGNATURE:
CARE GROUP: All in-patient children	DATE:

STANDARD
OBJECTIVE: Medicines are administered safely
RATIONALE: There are significant differences in the prescribing and administration of paediatric medication. It is essential that medicines are administered to children under the direction of a registered children's nurse

NOTE: This standard applies only to administration of medicines by nurses. We acknowledge and welcome the fact that in some wards older children/parents administer medicines.

STRUCTURE	PROCESS	OUTCOME
S1 Each ward has a copy of the recognised medicines policy	The nurse: P1 adheres to the recognised medicines policy	O1 each child receives medicines in the manner specified in the hospital policy: —at the correct time —in the correct dose —by the correct route

---

* This example comes from RCN 1994 Standards of Care Series Paediatric Nursing, 2nd edition. Scutari, Harrow.

S2 Each registered nurse has access to a copy of the UKCC advisory paper on the administration of medicines	P2 refuses to administer medicines from, and seeks immediate advice about, unclear or dubious prescriptions	O2 any adverse effects of medication are recorded
S3 Each ward has an up-to-date copy of a pharmaceutical index	P3 records the reason for the omission of any prescribed medicine	
S4 A pharmacist is available to give advice	P4 observes each child for the adverse effects of any medicines administered	
S5 Medicines are available in paediatric dosages	P5 reports and records any adverse effects of medication and takes appropriate action	
S6 A prescription chart is completed and available for each child	P6 regularly updates her knowledge and skills	

Example 2

Statement of best practice*

TOPIC: CHILD HEALTH SURVEILLANCE

INTRODUCTION: Child health surveillance comprises four universal interventions: an antenatal contact; a primary birth visit; a second postnatal visit; and a 2 year appraisal.

If, for any reason any Child and Family team member is unable to deliver care as set out, it is the responsibility of the individual team member to bring this to the attention of the Senior Community Nurse (Child and Family) and they, in turn, to bring it to the attention of the Local Health Services Manager (if unable to solve the problem themselves).

Each Senior Community Nurse (Child and Family) must use his/her professional judgement to decide whether, and how

---

* Submitted by Yvette Buttery, Lifespan Healthcare NHS Trust.

much, additional input is required by individual cases (over and above four universal interventions). When additional input is required, an action plan must be agreed between a designated member of the Child and Family Team and the family.

This statement should be used in conjunction with relevant Trust policies and where appropriate patient preference.

SUB TOPIC: Two year to two year three months health appraisal
Staff involved in the development of this statement of best practice (for the sub topic 2 year to 2 year 3 month Health Appraisal): Lead Practitioner (Child And Family Services); Practice Development Group Members; Child Protection Advisor; Quality Facilitator; Clinical Effectiveness and Audit Coordinator; Community Paediatricians

TARGET POPULATION: Families with children aged 2 years to 2 years 3 months

OBJECTIVE: To ensure that all children receive a health appraisal between the ages of 2 years and 2 years 3 months

IMPLEMENTATION DATE: 1 April 1998

REVIEW DATE: October 1998

EVIDENCE/REFERENCES: Hall Report 1996; Polny 1993
Structure
The following structures/tools will be required:
—a designated member of the Child and Family Team with relevant experience
—clinical setting or client's home (whichever is most appropriate)
—scales and mimetre
—toys, books, bricks, threading bricks, pencils, paper, cups and teapots (for imaginary play)
—personal child health record (PCHR)
—development questionnaire/checklist.

Process
The following provides information about recommended processes:
—an appointment should be arranged by a designated member of the Child and Family Team

—the venue should be prepared (if appropriate)
—the child's development should be assessed using the development review questionnaire/checklist in conjunction with discussion with the parent/carer.

Concerns of any nature should be discussed with the Senior Community Nurse (Child and Family) who will decide on what further action/referral/care is required.

Any further action/referral/care needed should be discussed with the parent/carer, organised and recorded on the Index Card and PCHR.

Outcome
The following are intended outcomes:
—All children between 2 years and 2 years 3 months will have a health appraisal.
—Child and family needs will be identified and further care/action plan will be discussed, organised and recorded.
—Any referrals needed will be made to the appropriate agencies.
—The family will be aware of how to access Child and Family services in the future.

A series of proformas for clinical audit

Standard Form		
Reference No: Topic: Location: Client Group: Reason for topic selection: Key references: Objective:	Staff member responsible: Implement-by Date: Audit by Date: Standard Review Date:	
STRUCTURE	PROCESS	OUTCOME

Measurement Tool			
Objective: Sample: Time Frame: Auditor(s): Date:			
TARGET GROUP	METHOD	CODE	AUDIT CRITERIA

Audit Record				
Objective: Sample: Time Frame: Auditor(s): Date:				
TARGET GROUP	OBSERVATIONS 1 2 3 4 5 6 7.......100	TOTALS Obs Y N	COMPLIANCE Expected Actual	COMMENTS

Audit Summary		
Reference No: Sub-topic: Objective: Sample: Time Frame: Auditor(s): Summary Date:		
ACTIVITY	FINDINGS	CONCLUSIONS

Action Plan			
Reference No: Topic: Objective: Plan Date:			
Identified Problem	Suggested Action	Staff Member Responsible	Time Period

Audit Report
rationale – *your reasons for choosing the topic*
evidence base – *the evidence on which your standard is based*
standard – *the standard against which you have compared practice*
involvement – *professional and patient groups involved*
implementation – *the steps you took to implement the standard*
methods – *audit tool, sample and data collection strategy*
results – *summary of data analysis and changes in practice*
cost – *an approximation of the direct costs involved in the project*
lessons learned – *summary of the impact of the project*
recommendations – *issues for the report's audience*
references – *referred to in section on evidence*

Example of a completed set of proformas

STANDARD

STANDARD REF: 002   IMPLEMENT BY: JULY 1999
TOPIC: HEALTH PROMOTION   AUDIT BY: OCTOBER 1999
SUB-TOPIC: IMMUNISATION   SIGNATURE:
CARE-GROUP: ALL INFANTS UNDER DATE: 4 JAN 1999
                6 MONTHS
KEY REFERENCE:

Objective: Every infant has access to immunisation against diphtheria, tetanus, pertussis, polio and haemophilus influenza (B) before they are 6 months old

STANDARD FORM

STRUCTURE	PROCESS	OUTCOME
S1 System for calling all infants for vaccination at 2, 3 and 4 months	P1 All parents are notified by clerical staff	O1 All infants are fully immunised by the age of 6 months
S2 Staff training is provided and covers:	P2 Non-attenders are followed up at home by a health visitor	O2 Non-attenders are visited at home by a health visitor
—communication of relevant information to parents	P3 Suitability for immunisation is established	O3 Anaphylaxis and other immediate reactions are managed safely
—administration of vaccine to infants	P4 Consent is obtained from parents	
—the management of anaphylaxis and other immediate reactions	P5 (a) Vaccines are stored and (b) reconstituted according to product information	O4 Parents bring their infants for the full course of vaccines
S3 Staff have access to:	P6 Parents are given a clear explanation of:	O5 Parents can state the purpose of immunisation
—supply of vaccine	—the purpose of immunisation	
—sterile needles and syringes	—the number of clinical visits necessary	
—designated refrigeration facilities	—any side-effects and how to manage them	
—product information leaflets	P7 Vaccines are administered as per local protocol	
—local protocol for administration		

AUDIT FORM

AUDIT OBJECTIVE: To establish what proportion of infants are fully immunised and discover reasons for any shortfall.

SAMPLE: Population of infants between 6 and 12 months, random 20% sample of child health records (100).

Equal number of immunisations to be observed (100). Total population of staff (80).

TIME FRAME: 2 weeks

AUDITOR(S): Sister Smith, Dr Guha

DATE: 4 March 1999

TARGET GROUP	METHOD	CODE	AUDIT CRITERIA
CLIENTS	Check Records	O1	According to child health records has the child been fully immunised?
STAFF	Ask	S2	Have staff attended immunisation training/update within the last 12 months?
STAFF	Observe	S3	Is there a local protocol for administration?
STAFF	Observe	S3, P5a P5b	Are vaccines stored correctly? Are vaccines reconstituted according to product information?
STAFF	Observe	P7	Are vaccines administered as per local protocol?
CLIENTS	Check Records	O3	Were incidents of anaphylaxis and other immediate reactions managed safely?
CLIENTS	Ask	O5	Can parents state the purpose of immunisation?

AUDIT RECORD

AUDIT OBJECTIVE: To establish what proportion of infants are fully immunised and discover reasons for any shortfall.

SAMPLE: Population of infants between 6 and 12 months, random 20% sample of child health records (10).
Equal number of immunisations to be observed (100). Total population of staff (80).

TIME FRAME: 2 weeks

AUDITOR(S): Sister Smith, Dr Guha

DATE: 4 September 1999

TARGET GROUP	CODE	OBSERVATIONS 1 2 3 4 5 6 7 8 9 10 etc.	TOTALS Obs Y	N	COMPLIANCE Expected	Actual	COMMENTS
CLIENTS	O1	Y Y Y N N Y Y N Y Y	70	30	100%	70%	Children not fully immunised are from travelling families, from one area.
STAFF	S2	Y Y Y N N Y Y N N N	40	40	100%	50%	Four part-time staff had not attended recent training.
STAFF	S3, P5a, P5b	Y Y Y Y N Y Y Y Y Y	99	1	100%	99%	Receptionist's lunch in vaccine fridge
		Y Y Y Y Y Y N Y Y Y	98	2	100%	98%	One vaccine reconstituted with normal saline instead of water for injection.
STAFF	P7	Y Y Y Y Y Y Y Y Y Y	80	0	100%	100%	
CLIENTS	O3	Y	1	0	100%	100%	Only one incident, managed safely.
CLIENTS	O5	Y Y N Y Y Y Y Y N Y	80	20	100%	20%	Two women did not speak English, no interpreter available.

AUDIT SUMMARY

AUDIT OBJECTIVE: To establish what proportion of infants are fully immunised and discover reasons for any shortfall.

SAMPLE: 500 children between 6 and 12 months, sample of 100, 80 clinic staff, 100 immunisations observed.

TIME FRAME: 2 weeks
AUDITOR(S): Sister Smith, Dr Guha
DATE: 10 October 1999

ACTIVITY	FINDINGS
COMPLIANCE	70% of infants received a full course of immunisation.
STAFF TRAINING	50% of staff had attended training in the last 12 months.
DEDICATED STORAGE FOR VACCINES	99% vaccines stored correctly. One lunch in drug fridge.
RECONSTITUTION OF VACCINES	98% reconstituted correctly.
ANAPHYLAXIS	One incident, managed safely.
COMMUNICATION WITH PARENTS	80% of parents could state the purpose of immunisation.

ACTION PLAN

OBJECTIVE: Every infant has access to immunisation against diphtheria, tetanus, pertussis, polio and influenza (B) before they are 6 months old.

AUDIT OBJECTIVE: To establish what proportion of infants are fully immunised and discover reasons for non-compliance.

IDENTIFIED PROBLEM	SUGGESTED ACTION
Travelling families and families on Chilblow estate are not attending clinics.	Contact health visitor responsible for travelling families to explore problems.
	Posters in family centre on Chilblow estate, local health visitors to follow up individual cases.
Part-time staff are missing training opportunities.	Liaise with staff concerned to discuss times to provide training compatible with their working patterns.
Sandwich in fridge	Practice manager will investigate price of small fridge for staff coffee room.
Communication with parents	Review language of information leaflets.
	Liaise with local Asian Women's Groups.

Standard Form

Reference Number: SCHE28
Topic: POST NATAL CARE
Sub-Topic: BREAST FEEDING
Client Group: POST NATAL WOMEN WHO WISH TO BREAST FEED

Implement By Date: 30/05/1996
Audit/Assessor Date: 30/06/1996
Signature (1): CHRIS HUMBLES
Signature (2): MIDWIFERY PRACTICE GROUP

Location: MB2

Standard Date: 30/05/1996

Rationale:

Standard Statement: EACH WOMAN RECEIVES INFORMATION, ENCOURAGEMENT AND SUPPORT TO INITIATE AND MAINTAIN BREAST FEEDING

Structure	Process	Outcome
S1 Midwife	P1 The midwife explains the principles of initiating and maintaining breast feeding	O1 Each woman is given information on the principles of initiation and maintenance of breast feeding
S2 Breastfeeding philosophy	P2 The midwife assesses the woman's needs with her and negotiates a plan of care	O2 Breast feeding is initiated within first hour of life
S3 Resource file – with written guidance for midwives	P3 The midwife assists the woman to breast feed within one hour of delivery	O3 Each woman has knowledge of equipment and its availability
S4 Breast feeding literature for women	P4 The midwife documents the time of feeding	O4 Each woman has a plan of care specific to her breast feeding needs

Structure	Process	Outcome
S5 Environment conducive to breast feeding	P5 The midwife ensures the woman's privacy	O5 Each woman has knowledge of support groups
S6 Care Plan	P6 The midwife selects appropriate equipment if necessary, i.e. breast pump	O6 A private environment is available
S7 Support Groups	P7 The midwife teaches the woman how to use the equipment and how to access it if necessary	O7 The infant is exclusively breast fed during establishment of breast feeding unless medically indicated
S8 Referral mechanisms for specialist needs	P8 The midwife informs the woman of the available support groups	O8 Documentation is complete
S9 Breast feeding equipment	P9 The midwife evaluates and documents all care given	
	P10 The midwife provides ongoing support and encouragement for the breast feeding woman	
	P11 The midwife promotes exclusive breast feeding unless medically indicated	

Audit Record

Reference Number: SCHE28
Sub-Topic: BREAST FEEDING
Audit Objective: TO ACHIEVE THE STANDARD
Client/Provider: POSTNATAL MOTHERS WHO WISH TO BREAST FEED
Sample:
Sample Context: 7 POSTNATAL WOMEN ON MB2
Time-Frame: ONE WEEK
Auditors: ALL STAFF
Form Date: Audit Date: 22/06/1998

Target	Method	Audit Criteria	Code	Totals	Expect.	Actual
THE WOMEN	ASK THE WOMEN	WERE YOU OFFERED INFORMATION ABOUT THE BENEFITS OF BREAST FEEDING ANTENATALLY?	1	Y: 5/7 N: 2/7	100%	71%
THE WOMEN	ASK THE WOMEN	POSTNATALLY?	2	Y: 7/7 N: 0/7	100%	100%
THE WOMEN	ASK THE WOMEN	WERE YOU OFFERED HELP TO INITIATE BREAST FEEDING? (Note to Auditor: if help not needed or wanted score N/A)	3	Y: 7/7 N: 0/7	100%	100%
THE WOMEN	ASK THE WOMEN	WAS YOUR BABY OFFERED THE BREAST WITHIN ONE HOUR OF DELIVERY? IF NO – PLEASE GIVE DETAILS	4	Y: 7/7 N: 0/7	100%	100%

			No.	Y/N	%	%
MIDWIVES	RECORDS	IS THE TIME OF THE FIRST FEED DOCUMENTED? (On the Partogram or Care Plan)	5	Y: 7/7 N: 0/7	100%	100%
WOMAN	ASK	IF YOUR BABY WAS UNABLE TO BREAST FEED DUE TO SPECIAL CIRCUMSTANCES, WERE YOU GIVEN HELP AND ADVICE TO START YOUR MILK SUPPLY? (Note to Auditor: Please specify special circumstances)	6	Y: 1/2 N: 1/2	100%	50%
WOMAN	ASK	DID YOUR BABY RECEIVE BREAST MILK ONLY? IF NO, PLEASE RECORD WHY. (Note to Auditor: If formula milk was given, please note how it was administered, e.g. spoon, teat or cup)	7	Y: 5/7 N: 2/7	100%	71%
MIDWIFE	YELLOW CARD	IF THE BABY RECEIVED FORMULA MILK, WAS THIS MEDICALLY INDICATED?	8	Y: 1/2 N: 1/2	100%	50%
WOMAN	ASK	DID YOU DEMAND FEED YOUR BABY? IF NO, PLEASE GIVE DETAILS	9	Y: 7/7 N: 0/7	100%	100%
WOMAN	ASK	DID YOU RECEIVE INFORMATION REGARDING BREAST FEEDING SUPPORT GROUPS?	10	Y: 6/6 N: 0/6	100%	100%
WOMAN	ASK	WERE YOU OFFERED PRIVACY IN WHICH TO BREAST FEED?	11	Y: 7/7 N: 0/7	100%	100%
WOMAN	ASK	HAVE YOU CONTINUED TO BREAST FEED? IF NO, PLEASE COMMENT	12	Y: 7/7 N: 0/7	100%	100%
MIDWIFE	ASK	IS IN-SERVICE TRAINING RELATED TO BREAST FEEDING AVAILABLE FOR ALL HEALTH PROFESSIONALS WITHIN THE MATERNITY UNIT?	13	Y: 6/6 N: 0/6	100%	100%

MIDWIFE	ASK	14	IS THERE A COPY OF THE FOLLOWING AVAILABLE FOR ALL STAFF TO ACCESS? NMG GUIDELINES FOR BREAST FEEDING, INFANT FEEDING	Y: 6/6 N: 0/6	100%	100%
MIDWIFE	ASK	15	INFANT FEEDING PHILOSOPHY?	Y: 6/6 N: 0/6	100%	100%
MIDWIFE	ASK	16	WERE BREAST FEEDING NEEDS CLEARLY REFLECTED IN THE CARE PLAN?	Y: 6/6 N: 0/6	100%	100%

Reference No: SCHE28
Audit Date: 22/06/1998

Audit Data

Code	Data	1	2	3	4	5	6	7	8	9	10	11	12	13	14	15	Comments
1	Logical	Yes	No	Yes	Yes	Yes	Yes	No									NO ANTENATAL CLASSES
2	Logical	Yes	Yes	Yes	Yes	Yes	Yes	Yes									
3	Logical	Yes	Yes	Yes	Yes	Yes	Yes	Yes									SECOND BABY DID NOT REQUIRE HELP
4	Yes	Yes	Yes	Yes	Yes	Yes	Yes	Yes									
5	Logical	Yes	Yes	Yes	Yes	Yes	Yes	Yes									CAESAREAN SECTION
6	Logical	Yes						No									BY CUP TOP UP AT
7	Logical	No	Yes	Yes	Yes	Yes	Yes	No									CAESAREAN SECTION
8	Logical	Yes						No									
9	Logical	Yes	Yes	Yes	Yes	Yes	Yes	Yes									
10	Logical	Yes	Yes	Yes	Yes	Yes	Yes	Yes									
11	Logical	Yes	Yes	Yes	Yes	Yes	Yes	Yes									
12	Logical	Yes	Yes	Yes	Yes	Yes	Yes	Yes									
13	Logical	Yes	Yes	Yes	Yes	Yes	Yes	Yes									
14	Logical	Yes	Yes	Yes	Yes	Yes	Yes	Yes									
15	Logical	Yes	Yes	Yes	Yes	Yes	No reply	Yes									
16	Logical	Yes	No reply	Yes	Yes	Yes	Yes	Yes									

ACTION PLAN

Reference Number: SCHE 28
Sub-Topic: BREAST FEEDING
Standard Statement: EACH WOMAN RECEIVES INFORMATION, ENCOURAGEMENT AND SUPPORT TO INITIATE AND MAINTAIN BREAST FEEDING
Audit Objective: TO ACHIEVE THE STANDARD
Plan Date: 05/09/1997

Identified Problem	Suggested Action	Staff Member Responsible	Time Period
Q1 70% Were you offered information about the benefits of breast feeding	To continue to educate and encourage women to attend antenatal classes.	All Staff/S Ginn	Ongoing
	As multigravida women do not attend classes, ensure all women have breast feeding leaflets, to discuss with clinical manager.	S Ginn	One week
Q6 50% If your baby was unable to breast feed due to special circumstances, were you given help and advice to start your milk supply?	Only one woman was not given any help. Possibly due to staff on duty unfamiliar with humilactor. Contact the representative of humilactor to demonstrate use to staff, including health care assistants. Identify if more humilactors or hand pumps are required.	S Ginn	Within three months
Q7 71% Did your baby receive breast milk only?	Encourage staff to advise the use of cup feeding, hand express, or use the humilactor. Discuss with the Breast Feeding Initiative Group the possibility of organised in-service training.	S Ginn	One month
Q8 50% If baby received formula milk was this medically indicated?	Of the seven women audited, five of the babies did not receive formula milk, one did after discussion with the paediatrician. It is important to document on care plan reasons for giving formula milk. At next ward meeting discuss record keeping.	S Ginn	Two weeks

Appendix 4

National Centre for Clinical Audit (NCCA) criteria for clinical audit

The purpose of the NCCA criteria for clinical audit is to provide guidance on good practice in clinical audit for practitioners carrying out clinical audits, local or national audit groups or committees, purchasers funding audit programmes, and others.

CRITERION	EXPLANATION
1. Stakeholders in a service contribute ideas for audits and are involved in the audit process as appropriate.	Patients or clients, carers, internal or external service users, and purchasers, as appropriate, are enabled to suggest topics for audit, directly or indirectly, to the individual or group responsible for audit in a service. Stakeholders also may suggest aspects of the quality of care or service to be included in an audit and may participate in the audit process as appropriate.
2. The topics selected for audit are important to the quality of care.	Important topics are those which involve one or more of the following: ■ A large number of patients or clients. ■ Higher than usual risk to patients or staff. ■ A concern about the quality of care raised by patients, carers, users, staff or purchasers. ■ Potential for improving the effectiveness of care or service. ■ A costly intervention or service or the potential to improve cost effectiveness.
3. One or more specific quality improvement-related objectives for an audit are stated	Objectives are defined clearly and are focused on achieving improvement in the quality of care or service. Objectives consider stakeholders' views as far as possible.

4. Explicit measures of one or more aspects of care or service are established to enable comparison between actual practice and good practice.

Explicit measures state clearly and unambiguously what is to be assessed about actual practice. They can be about any aspect of care or service that is relevant to the audit objectives, including: documentation or information; critical processes; clinical, educational, or behavioural outcomes; critical incidents; or adverse events.

5. The audit objectives and measures reflect the best available evidence of good practice.

The audit design reflects up-to-date, sound evidence of good practice. If research evidence is not available for a topic, the audit design reflects national or local consensus on good practice.

6. The number and type of cases to be included in an audit, and the time period over which they are to be drawn, are defined clearly and are appropriate to the audit objectives and measures.

The number of cases, episodes, or occurrences and how they are to be selected, including any to be excluded, are described before data are collected. If cases are identified for inclusion in an audit but are excluded subsequently, the reason is stated clearly.

7. Valid and reliable data are collected to enable a comparison between actual practice and good practice.

Audit data are valid if they relate directly to the agreed objectives and measures. Audit data are reliable if different people collecting data, or the same person collecting the same data at different times, make(s) the same or almost the same judgements about actual practice.

8. The collection and use of data meet accepted ethical principles and provisions for confidentiality.

If an audit involves collecting information directly from patients, carers, or staff, care is taken to ensure that the procedure for collecting data and the information recorded are consistent with accepted ethical principles. Audit data are collected, handled, and presented consistent with agreed confidentiality policies related to audit.

9. Data are analysed using appropriate methods.

The methods used for grouping data collected for an audit and the statistics used for analysis of the data provide a complete, accurate, and unbiased picture of actual practice.

10. Data are presented to show clearly the relationship of actual practice to the objectives.

The methods used for presenting the data help the audit group members to understand how actual practice compares with good practice (as defined by the measure used in the audit) and whether or not objectives for the audit are being met.

11. Formal evaluation of the data is carried out by the audit group to analyse the findings and to identify any shortcomings in the provision of care and their causes.

In the evaluation process, the members of the audit group:
- Compare actual practice with good practice
- Analyse cases, occurrences, or situations which are not consistent with the audit measures and decide if the lack of consistency is or is not clinically acceptable
- Identify problems in the provision of care and their causes.

12. Needed improvements in practice are identified by the audit group.

Improvements identified are related to the agreed audit objectives, reflect the audit group's analysis of causes of problems which are affecting care or services, and are consistent with recognised good practice.

13. An action strategy and an action implementation plan are developed to achieve needed improvements in practice.

The action strategy uses a variety of approaches, as needed, to achieve and maintain improvements. The action implementation plan includes:
– Specific steps to be taken to address causes of problems identified and to achieve the needed improvements
– Individuals who are named as responsible to carry out the action
– Deadlines for execution of actions
– How and when the effectiveness and efficacy of the action is to be assessed.

14. The action plan is implemented.

Evidence is available to confirm that the audit findings have been acted upon or to support reasons for lack of action. Stakeholders in an audit are informed about action planned or taken as part of an audit.

15. Data collection, analysis, evaluation, and action are repeated as many times as required to confirm that improvements needed to meet the desired level of quality have been achieved and sustained.

Repeat data collection is designed to assess the effects of the action taken on the achievement of needed improvements. Several cycles of audit may be required to achieve the desired level of quality. When the decision is made not to re-audit, the reasons are stated clearly; for example, the needed improvements in care have been achieved.

Appendix 5

Framework for assessment

(From: Walshe K, Spurgeon P. Clinical audit assessment framework: Birmingham: Health Services Management Centre, University of Birmingham, 1997.)

Project assessment framework

Assessment sections of the framework

	Section		Question/issue
1.	Reasons	1.1	Were the reasons for undertaking the audit project clearly and explicitly stated?
		1.2	Were the reasons for undertaking the audit project systematically examined before the project started to assess its priority?
		1.3	Did the reasons for undertaking the audit project include: (a) the high volume, cost or risk associated with the topic area; (b) the existence of evidence of a serious quality problem in the topic area; (c) the existence of evidence on the clinical effectiveness of patterns of practice or intervention; and (d) the likelihood of a significant and achievable quality improvement in the topic area?
		1.4	Were the reasons for undertaking the audit project discussed and agreed with those working in the services/areas to be audited?

2.	Impact	2.1	Did the project result in an agreed action plan which explicitly set out the changes to services/areas which had been agreed and how they were to be implemented, set a timescale for their implementation, and assign individual responsibility for each change?
		2.2	Did the project result in improvements in the quality of health care provided to patients and/or in patients' health outcomes? Can those improvements be described? Can those improvements be quantified? Can the cost consequences of those improvements be estimated?
		2.3	Did the project result in improvements in the health care process? Can those improvements be described? Can those improvements be quantified? Can the cost consequences of those improvements be estimated?
		2.4	Did the project result in improvements in the structure, culture, organisation or environment in which health care is provided? Can those improvements be described? Can those improvements be quantified? Can the cost consequences of those improvements be estimated?
		2.5	Did the changes introduced as a result of the project become permanent, embedded in clinical and organisational practices?
3.	Cost	3.1	What were the approximate direct costs of undertaking the audit project, including both clinician and audit staff time costs but excluding minor/negligible costs, overheads and the cost consequences of any changes resulting from the project?
4.	Objectives	4.1	Were the objectives of the audit project clearly and explicitly stated, in a form that allowed an assessment to be made of whether or not they were met?
		4.2	Did the objectives of the audit project address both the collection of information about the topic area and the implementation of changes resulting from that information?

5.	Involvement	5.1	Did the project involve or consult those involved in or providing the services being audited or with an important interest in those services, including both clinical and non-clinical staff?
		5.2	Did the project involve or consult those with the authority to sanction any changes that the project might recommend, particularly if they had resource consequences or implications for other services/areas?
6.	Use of evidence	6.1	Was an appropriate literature search undertaken to identify research findings of relevance to the topic area being audited (including secondary sources such as Cochrane Library etc.)?
		6.2	Were available research findings used appropriately within the audit project?
		6.3	Was appropriate use made of the experience of others from elsewhere in undertaking audit projects on the same or similar topics (e.g. using NCCA resources or similar)?
7.	Project management	7.1	Was a project plan developed, which explicitly set out the proposed activities to collect, analyse and act on data about the topic/area, set target dates for completion and assigned responsibility for tasks to individuals?
		7.2	Were proper records kept of the project as it progressed, sufficient to allow those involved to manage the project effectively and monitor its progress against the project objectives and plan?
8.	Methods	8.1	Were any tools or instruments used in data collection (e.g. forms, surveys, etc.) designed carefully, making good use of existing available instruments, and piloted or tested before use?
		8.2	In projects entailing the collection of quantitative data, was the number of cases for which data were collected determined in advance, based on calculations of the accuracy with which quantitative measures needed to be estimated?
		8.3	Was the data set collected clearly focused around the project's objectives and limited only to data that were likely to be relevant and useful?

9.	Evaluation	9.1	Was the project evaluated after it was completed by those who had been involved in selecting and undertaking the project?
		9.2	Were the objectives which were set at the outset of the project met?
		9.3	Was the impact of the project (detailed above) worthwhile given the costs of the project (also detailed above)?
		9.4	Were any significant problems encountered during the project, and were they successfully resolved?

Programme assessment framework

Assessment sections of the framework

1.	Topic identification and selection	1.1	Is there a systematic approach to identifying, prioritising and selecting topics for clinical audit in place and in use?
		1.2	As part of the process of topic identification, are available routine information systems and sources used to identify potential quality problems for consideration?
		1.3	Does the process of identifying, prioritising and selecting audit topics involve all appropriate stakeholders, such as clinicians (from all relevant professions) working in the department/service, managers within the organisation, purchasers, and clients/users?
		1.4	Does the prioritisation of potential audit topics take into account: (a) the high volume, cost or risk associated with the topic; and (b) the existence of evidence of a serious quality problem; and (c) the existence of evidence on the clinical effectiveness of patterns of practice or interventions; and (d) the likelihood of a significant and achievable quality improvement?

2.	Impact	2.1	Are there effective change management structures and mechanisms in place to ensure that the actions and recommendations resulting from clinical audit activities are implemented and that implementation is effectively monitored?
		2.2	Does the programme result in improvements in the quality of health care provided to patients and/or in patients' health outcomes? Can those improvements be described? Can those improvements be quantified? Can the cost consequences of those improvements be estimated?
		2.3	Does the programme result in improvements in the health care process? Can those improvements be described? Can those improvements be quantified? Can the cost consequences of those improvements be estimated?
		2.4	Does the programme result in improvements in the structure, culture, organisation or environment in which health care is provided? Can those improvements be described? Can those improvements be quantified? Can the cost consequences of those improvements be estimated?
		2.5	Have the changes introduced as a result of the programme become permanent, embedded in clinical and organisational practices?
		2.6	Is the programme well regarded and valued by stakeholders in clinical audit, such as clinical staff from different professional groups, provider organisation managers, purchaser organisations and patient/user groups?
3.	Cost	3.1	What are the approximate direct costs of the clinical audit programme, including both clinician and audit staff time costs but excluding minor/negligible costs, overheads, and the cost consequences of any changes resulting from clinical audit?
		3.2	Are the costs of the programme well controlled and managed, with the expenditure of all resources clearly focused on achieving the programme's aims and objectives?

Improvement sections of the framework

	Section		Question/issue
4.	Management and direction	4.1	Is overall responsibility for clinical audit placed with a single, senior clinician who has the necessary skills in and understanding of clinical audit, has time available to fulfil this responsibility, and practises clinical audit him/herself?
		4.2	Does the senior clinician with overall responsibility for clinical audit command the respect and support of his/her own and other clinical professions?
		4.3	Are senior managers and/or Board members genuinely involved in and committed to the clinical audit programme?
		4.4	Is there a coherent and well understood strategy for quality improvement linking the management and direction of the clinical audit programme to other quality improvement initiatives (such as risk management, the Patient's Charter, TQM/CQI, etc.)?
		4.5	Is there a group or committee responsible for directing the clinical audit programme which meets regularly and whose membership and attendance includes representatives of both a range of different departments/services and a range of different clinical professions?
5.	Planning	5.1	Is there a written strategy for clinical audit, which sets out the long-term aims and objectives of the clinical audit programme and the activities, structures and resources put in place to achieve those aims and objectives?
		5.2	Is there a forward plan for clinical audit, which is linked to an overall strategy for clinical audit and translates longer-term aims and objectives into shorter-term targets with set timescales, deadlines and assigned responsibilities?
		5.3	Are the forward plan for clinical audit and the strategy for clinical audit reviewed and updated periodically?
		5.4	Is there a system in place and working for developing and agreeing forward plans for clinical audit with individual departments/services?

6.	Support and resources	6.1	Is there a named individual responsible for managing the clinical audit programme for whom this is their sole or main responsibility?
		6.2	Does the person responsible for managing the clinical audit programme have the necessary skills in clinical audit, project management, and the ability to liaise with and advise senior clinicians and managers?
7.	Coverage and participation	7.1	Are there active audit groups or teams working in all departments/services, undertaking clinical audit projects and involving all relevant professions and interest groups?
		7.2	Can all departments/services demonstrate that they have an active programme of clinical audit in place?
		7.3	Do all departments/services have a meeting/forum at which audit topics are discussed, results presented, changes agreed and progress in implementing those changes monitored?
		7.4	Is there a named individual clinician in all departments/services who has responsibility for clinical audit, takes the lead in organising and directing the department/service's clinical audit activities and reports on their progress?
8.	Training and skills development	8.1	Is there an ongoing programme of training in clinical audit for clinical professionals, and is the available training used by members of clinical staff from different departments/services and different professions?
		8.2	Is the training in clinical audit evaluated through formal feedback from participants, and does that evaluation suggest that the training is regarded as useful and worthwhile?
		8.3	Do all new members of clinical staff receive information about and training in the clinical audit activities of the organisation as part of their induction or orientation?

9.	Monitoring and reporting	9.1	Is there a system in place for collecting key data about clinical audit projects and for monitoring audit activities in departments/services against their agreed forward plans?
		9.2	Is the information collected from monitoring audit activities reported to those responsible for managing and directing the clinical audit programme, as well as to senior managers and/or Board members?
		9.3	Where the information from monitoring suggests that problems exist in the clinical audit activities of departments/services are appropriate incentives and sanctions in place to address those problems and is action taken to remedy them?
10.	Evaluation	10.1	Is the programme periodically reviewed and evaluated explicitly by those responsible for its management and direction?
		10.2	Is the progress made towards the aims and objectives of the programme examined periodically, and action taken when progress has been slower than necessary?
		10.3	Is an assessment made of whether the impact of the programme (detailed above) is worthwhile given the costs of the programme (also detailed above)?

Appendix 6
Further reading

Research texts

Bell 1993 Doing your research project, a guide for first-time researchers in education and social science. Open University, Milton Keynes

Burns N, Grove S K 1993 Practice of nursing research, 2nd edn. Saunders, Philadelphia

Cormack D (ed) 1996 The research process in nursing, 3rd edn. Blackwell Scientific Publications, Oxford

Depoy E, Gitlin L N 1994 Introduction to research: multiple strategies for health and human services. Mosby, St Louis

Hicks C 1990 Research and statistics. Prentice Hall, London

Oppenheim A N 1992 Questionnaire design and attitude measurement, 2nd revised edition. Pinter, London

Polit D E, Hungler B P 1989 Essentials of nursing research. Methods, appraisal and utilisation. Lippincott, Philadelphia

Sapsford R, Abbott P 1992 Research methods for nurses and the caring professions. OUP, Buckingham

Change management texts

Bennis W, Benne K, Chinn R 1976 The planning of change. Holt, Rinehart & Winston, Orlando, Florida

Handy C 1992 Understanding organisations. Penguin Books, London

Lancaster J, Lancaster W (eds) 1982 Concepts for advanced nursing practice: the nurse as change agent. Mosby, St Louis

Nolan V 1987 The innovator's handbook. Sphere Books, London

Sadler P 1995 Managing change. Kogan Page, London

Senge P 1990 The fifth discipline. Doubleday, New York

Upton T, Brooks B 1995 Managing change in the NHS. Kogan Page, London

Index

Evaluation form

As a part of the RCN's commitment to quality improvement we need your feedback as users of the handbook. In order to upgrade this publication for future editions we would appreciate your taking the time to photocopy this form, complete it and send it to the address at the end.

CONTENT

Was the handbook easy to read?   ☐ yes ☐ no
Comments:
....
....

Was the handbook set out logically?   ☐ yes ☐ no
Comments:
....
....

Do any particular sections need improving?   ☐ yes ☐ no
Please specify:
....
....

Are there any major omissions in the handbook? ☐ yes ☐ no
Please specify:
....
....

USEFULNESS

How have you used the handbook?

As a reference text	☐
As an individual study guide	☐
As a group study guide	☐
Other	☐ ....

Which section of the handbook have you found most useful?

....
....

How have you used the handbook in your practice?

....
....
....
....

Did you use the 'time out' boxes?　　　　　☐ yes ☐ no
Comments:

....
....

Would you recommend the handbook to others in the following groups?

Nursing	☐ yes ☐ no
Medicine	☐ yes ☐ no
Professions allied to medicine	☐ yes ☐ no
Consumers	☐ yes ☐ no

Please add any further comments you may have either on the following page or on a separate sheet.

Thank you.

Please send your completed form to:

The Clinical Audit Handbook Evaluation
RCN Institute
Radcliffe Infirmary
Oxford
OX2 6HE

Alternatively you can fax it to 01865 246787 or email
clare.morrell@rcn.org.uk or gill.harvey@rcn.org.uk